The Structured Oral Examination in Anaesthesia

Practice Papers for Teachers and Trainees – Primary FRCA

This book is made up of questions and answers that closely simulate the Royal College of Anaesthetists' oral examination format. Set up as complete examination papers, the book enables candidates to assess their knowledge accurately and within time limits. The answers are presented thoroughly and clearly, with help from diagrams. Thorough revision of this book will be of benefit for anaesthesia oral examinations worldwide. The volume is an essential aid to study for trainees and a tool for trainers.

SHYAM BALASUBRAMANIAN is a Specialist Registrar at The Warwickshire School of Anaesthesia and The Heart of England Foundation Trust Hospitals in Birmingham. He is a Member of The Association of Anaesthetists of Great Britain and Ireland, and The Society for Intravenous Anaesthesia. He has practised anaesthesia in India, Canada and in the United Kingdom.

CYPRIAN MENDONCA is a Consultant Anaesthetist at the University Hospitals of Coventry and Warwickshire. He is a member of The Association of Anaesthetists of Great Britain and Ireland, The Obstetric Anaesthetists' Association and The Difficult Airway Society. Mendonca contributed a chapter to 'Core Cases in Obstetric Anaesthesia', published in 2004. He has practised anaesthesia in both India and in the United Kingdom.

COLIN PINNOCK is a Consultant Anaesthetist at Alexandra Hospital in Redditch, and an examiner for the Royal College of Anaesthetists. He has written and edited several market-leading textbooks including Fundamentals of Anaesthesia and has contributed to many more – such as the Qbase series.

The Structured Oral Examination in Anaesthesia

Practice Papers for Teachers and Trainees – Primary FRCA

Dr SHYAM BALASUBRAMANIAN MD FRCA
Specialist Registrar
Warwickshire School of Anaesthesia
England

Dr CYPRIAN MENDONCA MD FRCA
Consultant Anaesthetist
University Hospitals Coventry and Warwickshire
Coventry
England

Dr COLIN PINNOCK MBBS FRCA
Consultant Anaesthetist
Alexandra Hospital
Redditch
Worcestershire
England

CAMBRIDGE UNIVERSITY PRESS
Cambridge, New York, Melbourne, Madrid, Cape Town, Singapore, São Paulo

Cambridge University Press
The Edinburgh Building, Cambridge CB2 2RU, UK

Published in the United States of America by Cambridge University Press, New York

www.cambridge.org
Information on this title: www.cambridge.org/9780521680509

First published 2006

Printed in the United Kingdom at the University Press, Cambridge

A catalogue record for this publication is available from the British Library

Library of Congress Cataloguing in Publication data

ISBN-13 978-0-521-68050-9 paperback
ISBN-10 0-521-68050-6 paperback

Table of contents

Preface

I have been aware for some time that the amount of material aimed at candidates for the FRCA greatly outweighs that designed for trainers. There is so much good material available to revising candidates that there is really no excuse for sitting the examination inadequately prepared. Whilst this volume will hopefully help in revision terms, it is equally targeted at those worthy seniors who make themselves available for 'mock' oral examinations. I have used my experience of examining to ensure that the content of this book gives a representative feel for the real situation. Trainers wishing to conduct practice orals will find 10 ready-made structured examinations within. The format closely follows the current procedure of the primary FRCA and there are thus three topics to each subject – in line with current marking. Aspiring candidates will, I hope, also benefit from the revision material which is deliberately written in a semi-discursive style.

It is obviously imperative when training candidates about to sit the Royal College Examinations, that the subject matter is apposite. I hope those who read and use this book will appreciate the suitability of its content. Readers may care to note that the educationalist approved term for 'Viva' is now 'Structured Oral Examination' or SOE for short. This book therefore uses this parlance throughout.

My thanks are extended to my two co-authors, both of whom have played a large role in the organisation of the FRCA preparation courses at Coventry. Much of the material within has been used on these courses for some years.

Once again I wish those about to sit the examination good luck. Go well prepared!

Colin Pinnock
Alexandra Hospital
Redditch
April 2006

Acknowledgements

The authors thank Cambridge University Press for permission to use diagrams from Fundamentals of Anaesthesia 2nd edition. Thanks are also due to the original providers of these diagrams: Robert Jones, Ted Lin, Timothy Smith and Colin Pinnock. The authors gratefully acknowledge the support and help received from their colleagues.

Abbreviations

2,3-DPG	2,3 Diphosphoglycerate
5-HT	5 hydroxy tryptamine
A	Ampere
α	Alpha
ABG	Arterial blood gas
AC	Alternating current
ACEI	Angiotensin converting enzyme inhibitor
AChE	Acetyl cholinesterase
ACTH	Adrenocorticotrophic hormone
ADH	Anti-diuretic hormone
AMP	Adenosine mono phosphate
ANOVA	Analysis of variance
APL	Adjustable pressure limiting
APTT	Activated partial thromboplastin time
ARDS	Acute respiratory distress syndrome
ATP	Adenosine triphosphate
AV	Atrio-ventricular
β	Beta
BMI	Body mass index
BMR	Basal metabolic rate
BP	Blood pressure
BTPS	Body temperature pressure, saturated with water vapour
C	Celsius
Ca	Calcium
CBF	Cerebral blood flow
CNS	Central nervous system
CO	Cardiac output

COAD	Chronic obstructive airway disease
COMT	Catechol-O-methyl transferase
COX	Cyclo-oxygenase enzyme
CPAP	Continuous positive airway pressure
CPR	Cardio-pulmonary resuscitation
CRH	Corticotropin releasing hormone
CSF	Cerebro spinal fluid
CVP	Central venous pressure
CVS	Cardiovascular system
δ	Delta
Da	Dalton
DC	Direct current
DIC	Disseminated intravascular coagulation
DNA	Deoxyribonucleic acid
DVT	Deep vein thrombosis
ECF	Extra cellular fluid
ECG	Electrocardiogram
ECT	Electro convulsive therapy
EDTA	Ethylene diamine tetra acetic acid
EMG	Electromyogram
$ETCO_2$	End tidal carbon dioxide
ETT	Endotracheal tube
FADH	Flavine adenine dinucleotide (reduced)
FGF	Fresh gas flow
FRC	Functional residual capacity
FSH	Follicle stimulating hormone
γ	Gamma
GABA	Gamma amino butyric acid
GFR	Glomerular filtration rate
GH	Growth hormone
GIT	Gastro-intestinal tract
GnRH	Gonadotropin releasing hormone
GRH	Growth hormone releasing hormone
GTN	Glyceryl trinitrate
GTP	Guanosine triphosphate
H receptor	Histamine receptor
H	Hydrogen
Hb	Haemoglobin
HbF	Fetal haemoglobin

HbS	Sickle haemoglobin
HCO_3^-	Bicarbonate
HME	Heat and moisture exchanger
HPV	Hypoxic pulmonary vasoconstriction
HR	Heart rate
ICP	Intracranial pressure
Ig	Immunoglobin
IHD	Ischaemic heart disease
INR	International normalised ratio
IOP	Intra-ocular pressure
ISB	Isothermal saturation boundary
IV	Intravenous
J	Joule
K	Kelvin
L	Litre
LED	Light emitting diode
LH	Leutenising hormone
LMA	Laryngeal mask airway
LMWH	Low molecular weight heparin
LVEDP	Left ventricular end diastolic pressure
MAC	Minimum alveolar concentration
MAO	Mono-amine oxidase inhibitor
MAP	Mean arterial pressure
MH	Malignant hyperthermia
ml	Millitre
MRSA	Methicillin-resistant *Staphyloccocus aureus*
N	Newton
N_2O	Nitrous oxide
Na	Sodium
NADH	Nicotinamide adenine dinucleotide
NIBP	Non-invasive blood pressure
NMDA	*N*-methyl D-aspartate
NSAID	Non-steroidal anti-inflammatory drugs
P	Pressure
Pa	Pascal
PCO_2	Partial pressure of carbon dioxide
PEFR	Peak expiratory flow rate
PG	Prostaglandins
PIH	Prolactin inhibiting hormone

PO_2	Partial pressure of oxygen
PONV	Post-operative nausea and vomiting
PRH	Prolactin releasing hormone
PT	Prothrombin time
PTC	Post tetanic count
Q	Flow
R	Resistance
RAST	Radioallergosorbent test
REM	Rapid eye movement
RNA	Ribonucleic acid
RPF	Renal plasma flow
RQ	Respiratory quotient
RR	Respiratory rate
RS	Respiratory system
SD	Standard deviation
SEM	Standard error of mean
SNP	Sodium nitroprusside
SO_2	Oxygen saturation
STP	Standard temperature and pressure
SV	Stroke volume
SVR	Systemic vascular resistance
SVT	Supraventricular tachycardia
T_3	Tri-iodothyronine
T_4	Thyroxine
TBW	Total body water
TCI	Target controlled infusion
TIVA	Total intravenous anaesthesia
TOF	Train of four
TRH	Thyroid releasing hormone
TSH	Thyroid stimulating hormone
TT	Thrombin time
TXA	Thromboxane
UFH	Unfractionated heparin
UTP	Uridine triphosphate
V/Q	Ventilation–perfusion
VIE	Vacuum insulated evaporator
VMA	Vannilyl mandelic acid
WPW	Wolff–Parkinson–White syndrome

SOE 1

Physiology 1

Key topics: reflex arc, pituitary, ventilation–perfusion

Q1 Muscle spindles and the reflex arc

Can you tell me the components of the reflex arc?
The reflex arc is the basic unit of integrated reflex activity. It consists of a sense organ, afferent neuron, one or more synapses, an efferent neuron, and an effector.

What is the Bell–Magendie law?
In the spinal cord, dorsal roots are sensory (afferent neurons enter the spinal cord through the dorsal horn) and ventral roots are motor (efferents).

What is a monosynaptic reflex?
This describes the reflex occurring in a monosynaptic reflex arc. There is one synapse between afferent and efferent neurons. Example: knee jerk.

What is a polysynaptic reflex?
A reflex with more than one synapse. Example: withdrawal reflex.

What is the mechanism for the knee jerk?
Basically, it is a stretch reflex of quadriceps femoris (*stimulus*: tap on the tendon that stretches the tendon; *response*: muscle contraction).

What is the structure of a muscle spindle?
The muscle spindle consists of a group of muscle fibres enclosed in a connective tissue capsule, which is distinct from the rest of the muscle (embryonal in character and having less striations). These fibres are called *intrafusal* fibres. *Extrafusal* fibres are the regular contractile fibres of the muscle.

There are two types of muscle fibres:

- Nuclear bag fibre (containing many nuclei).
- Nuclear chain fibre (thinner and shorter).

There are two types of sensory innervations:

- Primary endings, group Ia afferent fibres; rapidly conducting.
- Group II afferent fibres (flower spray ending) which innervate the nuclear chain fibres. The efferent (motor) supply is via A γ-fibres and β-fibres.

What is the function of the muscle spindle?

The muscle spindle and its reflex connections constitute a feedback device that helps to maintain the muscle length. If the muscle is stretched, spindle discharge increases and reflex shortening of muscle occurs. If the muscle is shortened without change in γ efferent discharge, the spindle discharge decreases and muscle relaxes.

What is a dynamic response?

This is the response to rate of change, that is the signal transmitted during the change in muscle length. The nerves from nuclear bag endings (type Ia afferent) discharge more rapidly while the muscle is being stretched and less rapidly during sustained stretch.

What do you understand by the term 'static response'?

The nerve endings on the nuclear chain fibres discharge at increased rate throughout the period when the muscle is stretched.

What is the inverse stretch reflex? Can you name the receptor for this reflex?

The inverse stretch reflex is the relaxation of muscle in response to a strong stretch.

Up to a point, the harder the muscle is stretched, the stronger is the reflex contraction. When the tension becomes maximal, the contraction suddenly ceases.

The receptor is the Golgi tendon organ, located at the tendon–muscle junction.

Q2 Endocrinology

What are the functions of posterior pituitary?

The posterior pituitary produces two hormones, vasopressin (ADH) and oxytocin.

ADH governs water homoeostasis and oxytocin stimulates milk ejection and contraction of the uterus.

Describe the functions of anti-diuretic hormone (ADH).

- Increases the permeability of collecting ducts by an effect on the aquaporin 2 receptor so that water enters into the hypertonic interstitium of the renal pyramids.
- Vasoconstriction.

- Glycogenolysis in liver.
- Stimulation of clotting factor production.

What controls ADH secretion?

ADH is stored in the posterior pituitary. Secretion is mediated through osmoreceptors located in the anterior hypothalamus (they are located in circumvillate organs, outside the blood brain barrier).

Secretion is increased by reduced volume of extra cellular fluid (ECF), increased osmotic pressure, pain, emotion, stress, nausea, vomiting, and angiotensin II.

Secretion is decreased by low osmotic pressure, increased ECF volume, and alcohol intake.

What hormones are secreted by the anterior pituitary?

Adrenocorticotrophic hormone (ACTH), thyroid stimulating hormone (TSH), growth hormone (GH), follicle stimulating hormone (FSH), leutenising hormone (LH), and prolactin.

Can you explain how the hypothalamus controls anterior pituitary hormone secretion?

By a feedback mechanism mediated by chemical agents secreted by hypothalamus through the portal hypophyseal vessels which act on the anterior pituitary.

Name the hormones secreted by the hypothalamus.

These include both releasing and inhibiting hormones:

- Corticotropin releasing hormone (CRH).
- Thyrotropin releasing hormone (TRH).
- Growth hormone releasing hormone (GRH).
- Gonadotropin releasing hormone (GnRH).
- Prolactin releasing hormone (PRH).
- Prolactin inhibiting hormone (PIH).

Why they are called hypophysiotropic hormones?

Because they are directly carried from hypothalamus to the anterior pituitary by portal hypophyseal vessels.

What is a portal circulation?

A portal circulation is one that connects two capillary beds. It does not receive arterial supply and does not drain into a venous system.

Can you name two portal circulations in the body?

- Hepatic–portal circulation.
- Hypothalamic–portal circulation.

Q3 Respiratory physiology – ventilation–perfusion

Can you explain the distribution of blood flow within the lungs?

Blood flow within the lungs in mainly determined by the gravity. In an upright lung blood flow decreases linearly from bottom to top.

Tell me more about the distribution of ventilation within the lungs?

Intrapleural pressure is more negative in the top and less negative at the bottom of lung. This has influence on the alveolar size. The apex of the lung has a big resting volume and needs a large expanding pressure and results in a small change in volume in inspiration. The base of the lung is more compliant. Ventilation also decreases from bottom to top (but less than the blood flow).

Explain the significance of the West zones.

Zone 1: PA > Pa > Pv, ventilated and underperfused area, alveolar dead space.
Zone 2: Pa > PA > Pv, optimal ventilation–perfusion matching.
Zone 3: Pa > Pv > PA, perfused and underventilated area, shunt.
(PA: alveolar pressure; Pa: arterial pressure; Pv: venous pressure)

What is dead space ventilation?

It is the volume of fresh inspired gas that does not take part in gas exchange.

Dead space can be termed anatomical and alveolar. Anatomical dead space corresponds to conducting airways and alveolar dead space consists of parts of lung that are ventilated but not perfused. Physiological dead space is a combination of anatomical and alveolar dead space.

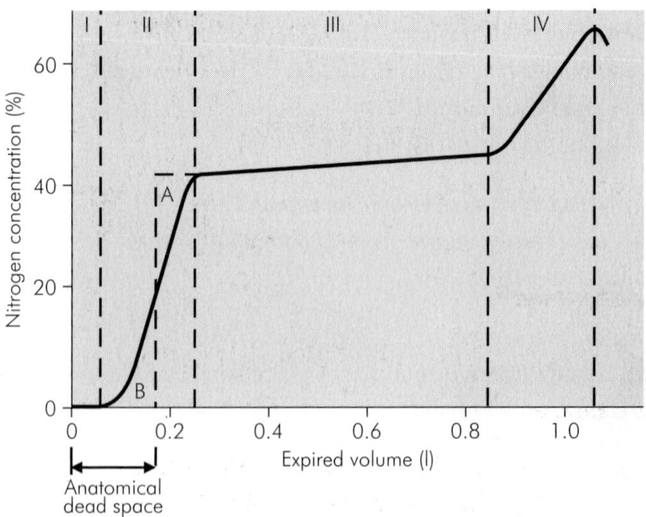

Figure 1.1 *Fowler's method of dead space measurement*

How do you measure anatomical dead space?

- By taking casts of conducting airways (historical).
- Fowler's method (single breath nitrogen wash out), non-invasively.

To begin with, the subject takes a single vital capacity breath of 100% oxygen and exhales through a nitrogen analyser. The concentration of expired nitrogen is plotted on the y-axis against the expired volume on the x-axis. Phase I represents the dead space gas that is free of nitrogen. Then gas from the alveoli starts mixing in the exhaled volume which is shown in phase II. Then an alveolar plateau is reached in phase III. To calculate the anatomical dead space phase II is divided by a vertical line so that area A = area B. The normal value is about 2 ml/kg.

How can you measure physiological dead space?

This is measured using Bohr's equation:

$$V_D/V_T = (P_aCO_2 - P_ECO_2)/P_aCO_2$$

E: mixed expired, a: arterial.

Can you derive Bohr's equation?

The principle behind Bohr's equation is that all the expired carbon dioxide (CO_2) comes from the alveolar gas.

$$V_A = V_T - V_D$$

alveolar volume is tidal volume minus the dead space. Therefore,

$$V_T = V_A + V_D$$
$$V_T \cdot F_ECO_2 = V_A \cdot F_ACO_2 + V_D \cdot F_ICO_2$$

But $F_ICO_2 = 0$. Therefore,

$$V_T \cdot F_ECO_2 = V_A \cdot F_ACO_2,$$

as discussed, now $V_A = V_T - V_D$

$$V_T \cdot F_ECO_2 = (V_T - V_D) \cdot F_ACO_2$$

expanding the equation

$$V_T \cdot F_ECO_2 = V_T \cdot F_ACO_2 - V_D \cdot F_ACO_2$$

rearranging the equation

$$V_D \cdot F_ACO_2 = V_T \cdot F_ACO_2 - V_T \cdot F_ECO_2$$
$$V_D \cdot F_ACO_2 = V_T (F_ACO_2 - F_ECO_2)$$
$$V_D/V_T = (F_ACO_2 - F_ECO_2)/F_ACO_2$$

Substituting partial pressure instead of concentration,

$$V_D/V_T = (P_ACO_2 - P_ECO_2)/P_ACO_2$$

P_ACO_2 may be taken as being equal to P_aCO_2 and hence,

$$\text{Dead space} = (P_aCO_2 - P_ECO_2)/P_aCO_2$$

F: fraction, A: alveolar, a: arterial, E: mixed expired, I: inspired, P: partial pressure.

Pharmacology 1

Key topics: agonist–antagonists, inhalation agents, anti-hypertensive drugs

Q1 Agonists–antagonists

What are agonists and antagonists?

- Agonists are those drugs that have receptor affinity and intrinsic activity.
- Antagonists have receptor affinity but no intrinsic activity.

What do you mean by affinity and intrinsic activity of a drug?

Affinity is 'how avidly a drug binds to its receptor'.

Activity (intrinsic efficacy) describes the 'magnitude of effect the drug has once bound'.

What are partial agonists? Can you give examples?

Partial agonists are drugs that have affinity, but limited intrinsic efficacy. Example: buprenorphine.

What is a dose–response curve? What is the shape of the curve?

A dose–response curve is a graphical plotting of concentration of the drug on the x-axis and the response on the y-axis. The shape is hyperbolic.

What is a log-dose–response curve? What is its advantage?

A log-dose–response curve is a semi-logarithmic plot with logarithm of the dose on the x-axis and response on the y-axis. Unlike the hyperbolic shape of the dose–response curve this is sigmoid shaped. The mid section of the curve approximates to linearity making the assessment of relation between dose and response easier to understand.

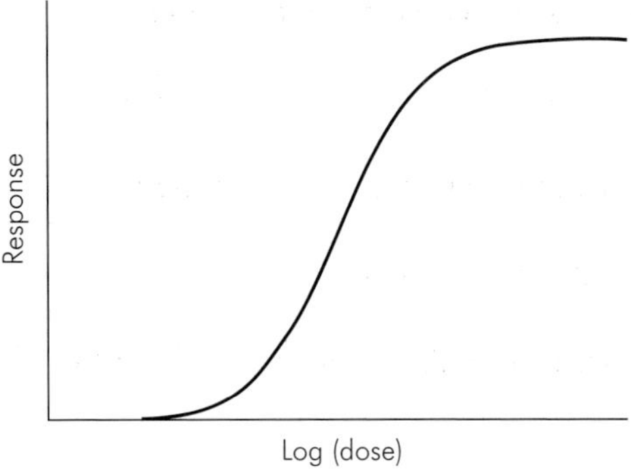

Figure 1.2 *Log-dose response curve*

What happens to the shape of the curve if the drug is a partial agonist?
Maximum response is reduced.

Draw me the effect of adding an antagonist on the dose–response curve?

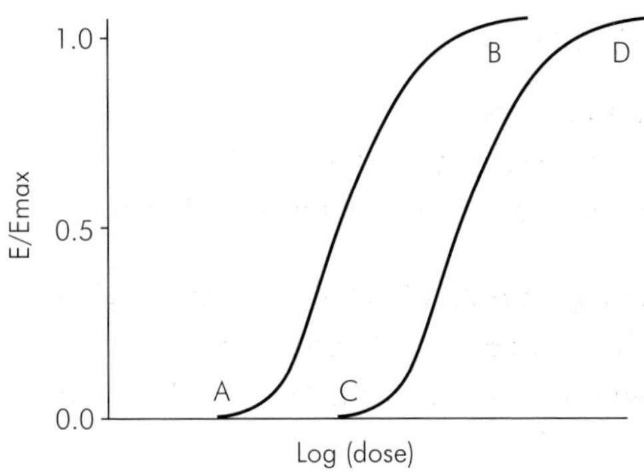

Figure 1.3 *Effect of adding an antagonist*

AB represents the curve of an agonist. CD represents the effect of adding a competitive antagonist. It is clear that more agonist is needed to achieve the same response. In the presence of a dose of non-competitive antagonist the curve is further shifted to the right and downwards. In other words, the maximum achievable response is reduced.

What types of 'antagonists' are you aware of? Give examples.
Antagonists are the drugs that bind to receptors with affinity but lack intrinsic activity and hence do not activate them. They can be:

- *Competitive*: In which case they bind reversibly with the receptor and displace the agonist. Higher doses of agonist can overcome this effect. Example: naloxone.
- *Non-competitive*: These agents will bind irreversibly with the receptors. Even increasing the dose of agonist cannot reverse this effect if the non-competitive antagonists are in high concentration. Example: phenoxybenzamine.

- *Physiological*: The agonist and antagonist act at different receptors but produce opposing effects. Example: epinephrine and histamine.

What is the difference between a competitive antagonist and an inverse agonist?

Competitive antagonists have no direct effect of their own but prevent an agonist having effect. Example: acetylcholine and atracurium at the neuro-muscular junction. Inverse agonists have opposite effects to the natural agonist. Example: acetylcholine and atropine at muscarinic receptors.

Q2 Inhalation agents

Can you describe the properties of an 'ideal inhalation agent'?

Break up the answer as follows:

- *Pharmaceutical properties*:
  - Liquid at room temperature
  - Chemically stable (light, heat, soda-lime)
  - Long shelf life, no additive
  - Non-irritant, pleasant smell
  - High saturated vapour pressure (for easy vaporisation)
  - Low latent heat of vaporisation
  - Low specific heat capacity
  - Inexpensive
  - Environmental friendly
- *Pharmacokinetic properties*:
  - Low blood/gas solubility
  - High oil/water solubility
  - Minimal metabolism
- *Pharmacodynamic properties*:
  - Smooth, rapid induction
  - Bronchodilatation, no respiratory depression
  - No cardiovascular depression/sensitisation to catecholamines
  - Analgesic, anti-emetic, anti-convulsant
  - Muscle relaxation
  - No increase in cerebral blood flow/intracranial pressure
  - No adverse hepatic, renal, haematological effects
  - Non-trigger for malignant hyperthermia
  - No effects on uterus
  - Not teratogenic/carcinogenic

What properties of an inhalation agent determine the onset and potency?

Onset: blood/gas solubility (lower → faster)

Potency: oil/gas solubility (higher → potent)

What inhalation agents do you use in your day-to-day practice?

Isoflurane, sevoflurane, desflurane.

How do isoflurane/sevoflurane comply with the criteria for an 'ideal inhalation agent'?

Best described by drawing a comparison table.

Table 1.1 *Isoflurane and sevoflurane*

Property	Isoflurane	Sevoflurane
Thymol required	No	No
Stable in light	Yes	Yes
Sodalime	Safe	Compound A
Cost	+	++
SVP (kPa)	33	22
Minimum alveolar concentration (MAC)	1.16	2
Blood gas co-efficient	1.4	0.69
Oil gas co-efficient	97	53
Irritant to breathe	+	–
Cardiac output/systemic vascular resistance (SVR)	↓	↓
Sensitivity to catecholamines	+	–
Metabolism percentage	0.2	3–5
Safety in pregnancy	++	?
Malignant hyperthermia (MH) potential	+	+

+: positive effect, –: no effect, ↓: decrease, ?: not known.

Q3 Anti-hypertensive drugs

Can you give a classification of anti-hypertensives? Tell me where they act.

Anti-hypertensives can be classified based on their site of action:

1 *Centrally acting*: Clonidine, methyl dopa.

2 *Heart*: Beta-blockers: atenolol.

3 *Vasodilators*:

- Angiotensin converting enzyme inhibitor (ACEI): captopril.
- Angiotensin antagonists: losartan.
- Calcium channel blockers: nifedipine.
- Alpha Blockers: prazosin.
- Nitric Oxide formation: sodium nitropruside (SNP), glyceryl trinitrate (GTN).
- Ganglion blocking drugs: trimethaphan.

4 *Kidney*: diuretics, thiazides.

Tell me some complications of ACEI.

Dry cough (↑ bradykinin in lungs); angio-edema, neutropenia, and renal failure in bilateral renal artery stenosis.

What are the problems in using SNP?

- SNP is unstable in solution and needs to be protected from light.
- Compensatory tachycardia.
- Rebound hypertension following cessation of infusion.
- Increase in intracranial pressure due to cerebral vasodilatation.
- Impairment of hypoxic pulmonary vasoconstriction worsening V/Q matching.
- Cyanide toxicity (maximum dose 8 μg/kg/min); [each molecule of nitroprusside undergoes non-enzymatic degradation within the red cells to contribute five cyanide ions. Within acceptable maximal dose and normal liver function the cyanide ions are eventually metabolised in the presence of hepatic mitochondrial enzyme, rhodanase to non-toxic compound, thiocyanate which is excreted in urine. Infants can lack this enzyme making SNP unsafe in them].

Discuss the management of cyanide toxicity.

- *General measures*: Airway, breathing and circulation, oxygen.
- *Chelating agent*: Dicobalt edetate combines with cyanide to form inert compounds.
- *Sodium thiosulphate*: Converts cyanide to thiocyanate which is non-poisonous and water soluble which is excreted in urine.
- *Sodium nitrite*: Converts haemoglobin to methaemoglobin, which in turn binds with cyanide to form cyanmethaemoglobin.
- *B_{12} (hydroxycobalamin)* forms cyanocobalamin with cyanide.

List the indications for the use of beta-blockers in the peri-operative period.

- Chronic anti-hypertensive treatment.
- Ischaemic heart disease.
- Attenuation of laryngoscopic response.
- Anxiety.
- Thyrotoxicosis.
- Phaeochromocytoma.
- Hypotensive anaesthesia.

Beta-adrenergic blockers have been conventionally considered as a contraindication for patients with cardiac failure. Recent studies show that beta-blockers with intrinsic sympathomimetic activity have actually improved outcome in these patients.

How do beta-adrenergic blocking drugs act?

They are competitive antagonists at beta-adrenoceptors.

What are the various mechanisms by which these drugs reduce blood pressure (BP)?

The initial drop in BP is due to a fall in cardiac output. With continued treatment, by an unknown mechanism, the cardiac output returns to normal but BP remains low. They also act by:

- Resetting baroreceptor activity.
- Inhibition of the renin–angiotensin system.
- Pre-synaptic inhibition of noradrenaline release.

How can you classify beta-blocking drugs? Give examples.

- *Receptor selectivity*: beta-1 and beta-2 selectivity influence the side effect profile. Example: atenolol, metoprolol are cardioselective beta-adrenergic blockers, propranolol is non-selective.
- *Intrinsic sympathetic activity*: the drugs in this group have partial agonist activity at beta-adrenergic receptors. They may be useful in mild cardiac failure. Example: acebutolol, oxprenolol, and pindolol.
- *Membrane stabilising activity*: These agents have anti-arrhythmic activity. Example: labetolol.
- *Duration of action*: long acting (propranolol). Short acting (esmolol).

What are the side effects of beta-blockers?

- Provocation of bronchospasm.
- Cardiac failure.
- Heart block.
- Mask signs of hypoglycaemia in diabetics.
- Cold extremities, worsening peripheral vascular disease.
- Fatigue, depression and sleep disturbances.

Clinical 1

Key topics: asthma, laparotomy, latex allergy, anaphylaxis

Q1 A 46-year-old female is booked for urgent laparotomy for intestinal obstruction. Her past medical history includes asthma with several hospital admissions in the past for the same.

How will you manage this patient prior to surgery?

Detailed pre-operative assessment to include history from the patient, review of medical and nursing records and clinical examination. The likely problems with this patient include dehydration, electrolyte imbalance, acid base imbalance, asthma and compromised respiratory function as result of abdominal distension.

On clinical examination you elicit following clinical findings

- ***Patient looks ill, tired, and dehydrated***
- ***Abdomen distended, nausea and vomiting +***
- ***Urine output 10–20 ml/hour***

What other information do you want?
Need to check her BP, heart rate, state of peripheral perfusion (capillary refill), fluid balance (composition and quantity of intravenous fluids given). Check her respiratory rate, auscultate her chest for wheezes. Monitor oxygen saturation using pulse oximetry.

BP is 90/42 mmHg, HR is 110/min, RR is 22/min, bilateral extensive wheezes present, SpO_2 is 90% on room air.

What investigations you would like to do at this stage?
Full blood count, urea and electrolytes, blood glucose, electrocardiogram (ECG), Chest X-ray, peak expiratory flow rate (PEFR), and arterial blood gas analysis:

- ***Na^+ 132 mmol/l, K^+3.1 mmol/l***
- ***Urea: 9.3 mmol/l, Creatinine: 122 μmol/l***
- ***PEFR: 150 l/min***

The surgeon insists that she needs to go to theatre immediately as he has some other commitment later. Are you happy to anaesthetise now? Why?
No, her hydration needs to be addressed and her respiratory parameters need to be optimised.

How will you assess dehydration?

- *Vital signs*: Tachycardia, hypotension.
- *End organ perfusion*: Altered mental state, decreased urine output, and reduced skin turgor.

What electrolyte abnormalities does she have and what do you think is the cause?
Hyponatraemia and hypokalaemia. It is possibly due to vomiting and sequestration in the intestine.

How will you optimise her fluid status?
Intravenous fluids as guided by clinical parameters and monitoring. Initially Hartmanns with additional potassium would be indicated.

Admitting her to a High Dependency Unit and more invasive monitoring (like CVP) will be beneficial in pre-optimisation.

What are the types of IV fluids you are aware of?

Fluids can be given for:

- Maintenance
- Replacement
- Resuscitation

Grossly two types of fluids are available, crystalloids and colloids.

Compare and contrast crystalloids and colloids.

Table 1.2 *Crystalloids and colloids*

Crystalloids	Colloid
Salt or sugar containing solutions	Suspension of particles rather than a true solution
Freely cross biological membranes	Unable to cross or slowly cross semipermeable membranes
Only a fraction of administered volume remains in circulation	Mostly remains in circulation
Initial expansion of vascular compartment due to volume infused	Plasma expanders as water is drawn into the vascular compartment due osmosis
Generally safe	Risk of hypersensitivity reaction and impairment of coagulation
Ideal for replacing ECF losses	Ideal for replacing plasma/blood losses
Inexpensive	Expensive

What are the ways to give parenteral potassium supplementation? How fast can you correct? What precautions will you take?

Potassium chloride should be added to a one litre bag at a concentration of 20–40 mmol/l given slowly over of 4–6 h. Higher concentrations of potassium chloride may be given in severe depletion. In an intensive care setting potassium is given in more concentrated form (1 mmol/ml) through a central line. Highly concentrated solutions given peripherally can cause vascular necrosis.

Monitor ECG during infusion. As potassium is an important ion in the maintenance of membrane potentials and action potential, inadvertent administration of potassium can lead to life-threatening arrhythmias including ventricular fibrillation.

Why are you concerned about hypokalaemia?

- *Cardiovascular system*: arrhythmias.
- *Nervous system*: Muscle weakness, increased sensitivity to non-depolarising neuromuscular blocking drugs, and delayed recovery.

- *Gastrointestinal system*: paralytic ileus.
- *Metabolic alkalosis.*

What are the ECG changes in hypokalaemia?

Prolonged PR, flattened T-wave, T-wave inversion, prominent U-wave.

How will you assess the severity of asthma in this patient?

- *History*: Duration, functional limitation, previous hospital admissions.
- *Examination*: General and respiratory system.
- *Investigation*: PEFR, SpO_2, arterial blood gas (ABG), Chest X-ray (as directed by clinical presentation).

What drugs are used in the treatment of asthma?

Beta-2 agonists, anti-cholinergics, steroids, aminophylline, and magnesium (and of course, oxygen).

How can you improve her respiratory function?

- Nebulisation and antibiotics if there is co-existing infection.
- Good pain relief.
- Early involvement of physiotherapist and breathing exercises.

Comment about her PEFR. How can it be used to assess responsiveness to medication?

Her peak expiratory flow rate is significantly reduced. About 15% improvement following bronchodilator therapy implies the responsiveness to treatment.

Q2 Critical incident: high airway pressure

After induction and intubation you observe that the peak airway pressure goes up. It is 60 cmH_2O. When you tried to hand ventilate the bag is very tight.

What will you do?

Recognise that this is an inappropriately high peak airway pressure. Call for help and in the mean time take measures to handle the situation.

100% oxygen, Look at monitors for other vital parameters (ECG, SaO_2, $ETCO_2$, NIBP).

Finding the cause and managing the situation should be simultaneous.

ABC approach can be modified here. Check the circuit from machine up to endotracheal tube (ETT) in a logical manner. If necessary change on to a totally new circuit (Waters' bag fed from a cylinder, for example, in order to be sure that there is no equipment fault). Remember the recent cases of plastic debris in filters, etc. Separate out patient factors from equipment ones. Above all, bag manually and auscultate the lungs. List the differential diagnosis and treat each one in an appropriate manner.

Give me some differential diagnoses.

- Wearing off of paralysis.
- Bronchospasm (asthma, anaphylaxis).
- Tension pneumothorax.
- Endotracheal tube in main bronchus.
- Obstruction, kinking, etc.
- Circuit obstructions.

Q3 Latex allergy

Assume the bronchospasm is due to a latex allergy. What are the predisposing factors?

Usually occurs in persons who get repeated exposure to latex. Example: health workers, patients exposed to repeated bladder catheterisation, patients who have occupational exposure to latex, patients with history of anaphylaxis of uncertain aetiology. Often there is history of atopy, cross allergies to chestnuts/banana, etc.

How does latex allergy present?

Its presentation can fall anywhere in the spectrum ranging from simple contact dermatitis to life-threatening anaphylaxis.

Can you explain the mechanism of these reactions?

Contact dermatitis is a type IV delayed hypersensitivity reaction, mediated by T-lymphocytes. It is probably a reaction to the anti-oxidants and stabilisers used in the manufacturing process of latex rubber.

Life-threatening anaphylaxis is a type I hypersensitivity reaction, occurring in latex sensitised individuals on re-exposure to the antigen (latex). Latex proteins cross link with the IgE antibody, lead to mast cell degranulation. This releases histamine, leukotrienes and prostaglandins and these result in profound vasodilatation, myocardial depression and bronchospasm.

If a known case of latex allergy comes to the theatre what precautions should you take?

- Should be placed first on the operating list.
- Premedication with anti-histamines (chlorpheniramine, ranitidine), corticosteroids.

- Theatre needs thorough cleaning prior to this case (unoccupied for at least 2 h).
- Ensure full awareness of all staff involved with the patient.
- Latex free box (equipments, synthetic gloves, etc.).
- Having a database of latex free equipment.
- Induce in the operating theatre.
- Clear, visible signs on doors to theatre.
- Availability of resuscitative drugs and equipments to manage anaphylaxis.

Describe the management of anaphylaxis.

Immediate management:

- Stop administering the possible offending agents.
- Airway breathing circulation, 100% O_2.
- Epinephrine 0.5–1.0 ml of 1:1000 im or 0.5–1.0 ml of 1:10,000 i.v. slowly.
- Intravenous fluids.
- Secondary treatment: anti-histamines, corticosteroids.
- Inotropic/vasopressor support as needed.
- Bicarbonate therapy as guided by blood gas analysis.
- Blood sample for mast cell tryptase should be taken (1) after treating the reaction as soon as possible (2) About 1 h after the reaction and (3) 6 h after reaction. Elevated serum tryptase after an anaphylactic reaction indicates mast cell degranulation.

Later, all the events should be documented. The patient should be tested for an adverse drug reaction. Once the drug responsible for the event is identified, patient and the general practitioner should be informed in writing. After discussion with the patient, medic alert bracelet should be arranged. The event should also be reported to the Committee on Safety of Medicines.

How would you investigate for the suspected drug or causative agent for anaphylaxis?

Patient should be referred to the immunologist with complete details of the drugs given during the event and full description of the event.

Skin prick testing is the most commonly performed test (a drop of diluted drug solution is placed over the forearm skin, and then skin is punctured using a small gauge needle).

Occasionally intradermal testing using more dilute solution may be required. The skin tests are usually carried out 4–6 weeks after the reaction.

Radio-allergo absorbent test (RAST) is an alternative investigation. As it is performed in vitro, there is no risk of anaphylactic reaction during the test. It is less sensitive than a skin test and more expensive.

Physics, clinical measurement and safety 1

Key topics: humidification, capnography, filters

Q1 Humidification

Define water vapour pressure.

It is the pressure that would be exerted by water vapour if it alone occupied the space. It is expressed as kPa.

What do you mean by the term saturated water vapour pressure?

It is the maximum attainable water vapour pressure at a given temperature.

(*Note:* The maximum amount of water vapour that can be present in a given volume of air is determined by the temperature.)

What is absolute humidity?

Absolute humidity is the mass of water vapour present per unit volume of gas (mg/l or g/m^3).

What is relative humidity?

Relative humidity is the ratio of the mass of water vapour in a given volume of air to the mass required to saturate that given volume of air at the same temperature.

It is also expressed as (actual vapour pressure/saturated vapour pressure).

Define dew point.

Dew point expressed in °C is the temperature at which condensation occurs when the gas is cooled.

What does BTPS stand for? What is the isothermic saturation boundary (ISB)?

Alveolar gas is said to be at BTPS conditions (i.e. **b**ody **t**emperature and **p**ressure, **s**aturated with water vapour). Gas conditions are constant and therefore gas exchange is efficient.

The moisture deficit is the difference between 44 g/m^3 (the absolute humidity when gas in the alveoli is saturated with water vapour at 37°C) and the absolute humidity of inspired air. It is the humidity that must be added by the upper airways to condition the inspired air for optimal gas exchange in the alveoli.

The level in the airways where the gas reaches BTPS is the ISB.

What determines the ISB level?

Normally it is just below carina but its position varies according to the volume, temperature and humidity of the inspired gases and with tracheal intubation, which bypasses the upper airway.

It lies further down the airway as the volume increases, temperature and humidity decrease and after endotracheal intubation.

During inspiration air is heated and humidified so that its temperature and relative humidity increase as gas passes down the upper airway. Much of the heat and moisture exchange takes place in the nose, where heat and moisture of expired gases is conserved.

Classify humidification equipment. Give examples.

Humidification can be active or passive.

- *Active*: Adds water vapour to a flow of gas independent of the patient. Example: heated humidifiers, nebulisers.
- *Passive*: Returns a portion of the exhaled moisture or rely on a chemical reaction with exhaled CO_2 to humidify the expired gas. Example: heat and moisture exchangers (HME), circle absorbers.

Describe how HMEs function.

HMEs consist of a layer of either foam or paper that is generally coated with a hygroscopic salt such as $CaCl_2$.

The expired gas cools as it passes through the device and condensation occurs, releasing the massive enthalpy of vaporisation to the HME layer. The hygroscopic salt reduces the relative humidity of the gas to below saturation level by chemically combining with the water molecules, although some water vapour is lost into the breathing system.

On inspiration, the absorbed heat evaporates the condensate and warms the gas. The hygroscopic salt, to which the water molecules are loosely bound, releases the water molecules when the water vapour pressure is low.

The inspired gas is therefore warmed and humidified to an extent that depends on the moisture content of the expired gas, and hence on the patient's core temperature and the condition of the airways and lungs.

What is the efficiency of HME humidifiers?

With HME a relative humidity of 60–70% is achieved. The efficiency of the system declines over time and a filter is recommended only for a maximum period of 24 h.

What are the potential problems with their use?

- Add dead space that can cause increase in $PaCO_2$ unless total ventilation is increased to compensate.
- Increased resistance to gas flow. This may affect patient's ability to wean from mechanical ventilation and may affect the triggering of some ventilators. May be particularly marked if liquid (e.g. condensation or secretions or nebulised drugs) enters the HME.

- Efficiency depends on inspired tidal volume and minute volumes – less efficient at high minute volumes.
- Risk of infections with organisms such as *pseudomonas.*

Q2 Capnography

What is the principle behind capnography?

A capnograph uses the principle of infrared absorption by CO_2. Gases with molecules containing two or more different atoms absorb radiation in the infrared region of spectrum. CO_2 has a strong absorption band at a wavelength of 4.26 μm.

Draw a normal capnograph trace.

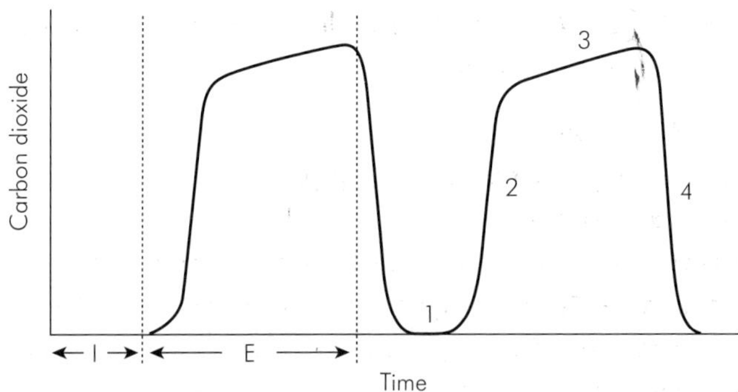

Figure 1.4 *Capnograph graph (I = inspiration, E = expiration)*

The phases of the normal waveform are as follows:

1 *Inspiration: This should be at 0, since any elevation of the baseline indicates rebreathing.*
2 *Upslope phase: Onset of expiration. If this is shallow it indicates obstruction.*
3 *Plateau: This represents mixing of alveolar gas; if sloped rather than flat, indicates uneven mixing, as in COAD (Chronic obstructive airway disease).*
4 *Fall to 0, Inspiratory downstroke.*

Where will you see the following capnograph traces?

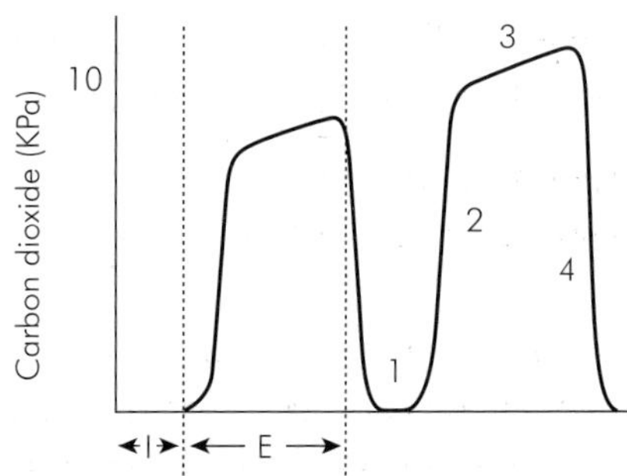

Figure 1.5 *MH: high plateau CO_2 – rapid rate*

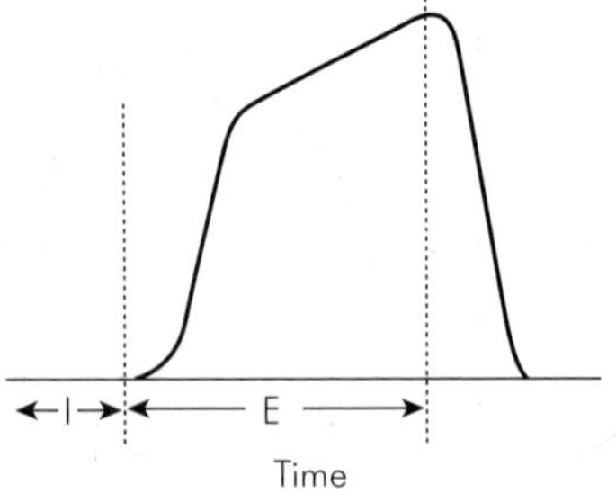

Figure 1.6 *COAD: Slow upstroke – sloping plateau wide $P(a\text{-}ET)CO_2$ gradient*

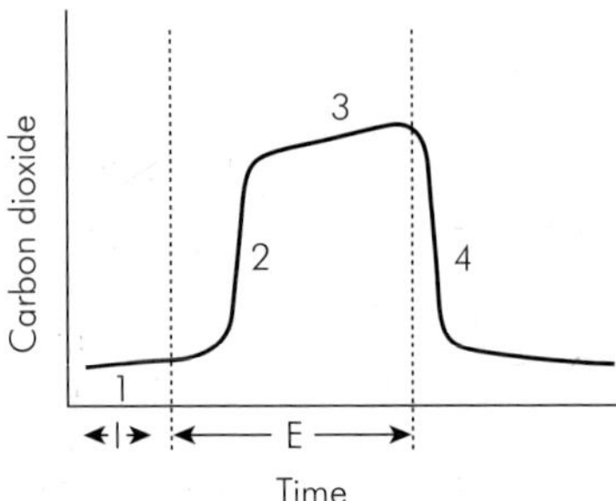

Figure 1.7 *CO_2 rebreathing – raised baseline*

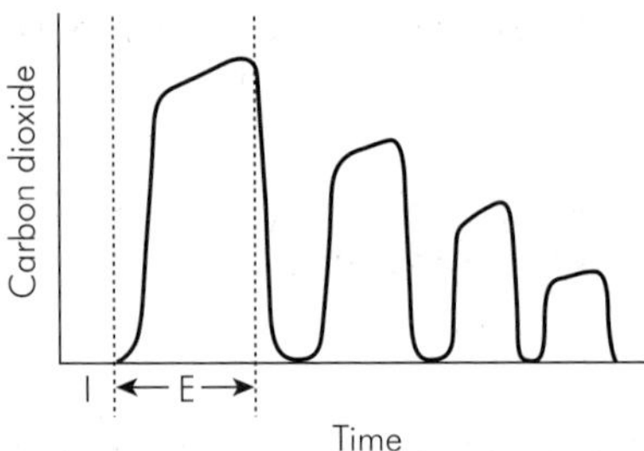

Figure 1.8 *Reduced cardiac output – progressive diminution in amplitude*

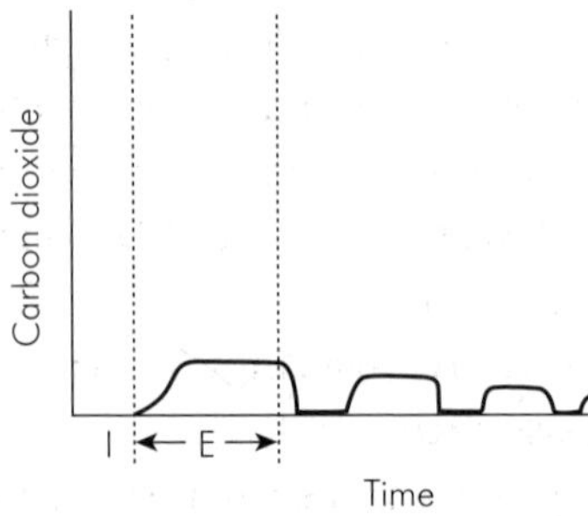

Figure 1.9 *Oesophageal intubation – even with carbonated drink in stomach, <6 deflections seen. Thereafter the ETT cannot be in the trachea unless circulatory arrest has occurred*

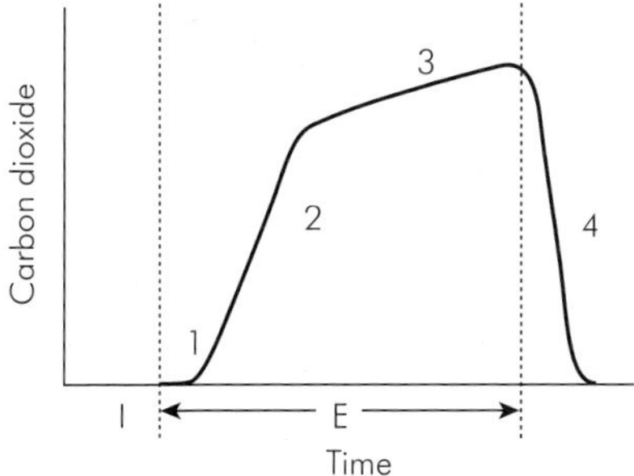

Figure 1.10 *Airway obstruction – slow ascent phase 2*

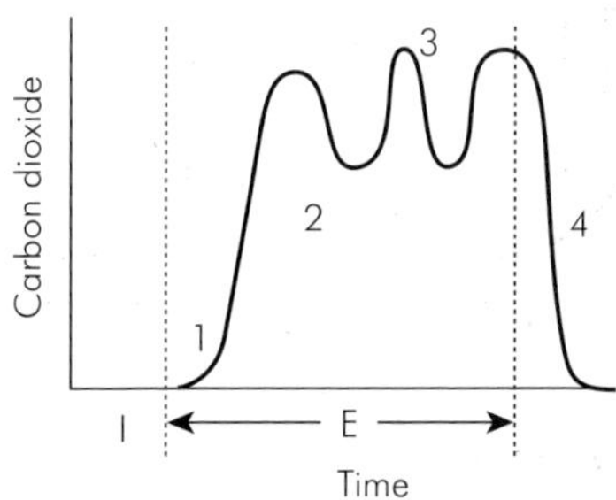

Figure 1.11 *Recovery from neuro-muscular blockade – clefts seen during phase 3*

How does a capnograph work?

A CO_2 analyser has three basic components:

- Infrared radiation source.
- Infrared photodetector.
- Two chambers, one for sampling and other for reference. Each chamber has about 1–2 ml volume.

The amount of infrared radiation absorbed is proportional to the CO_2 concentration. The electrical output from the photodetector is presented as a partial pressure of CO_2 in the sample chamber. The absorption detected from the sample chamber is compared with that from the reference chamber and precise estimation of CO_2 concentration is obtained. Using this technique CO_2 measurement is made continuously throughout respiratory cycle.

Depending on the location of the sampling chamber a capnograph can either be a main stream analyser or side stream analyser.

Main stream analysers give a relatively fast and accurate response. They are expensive, increase dead space and weight in the circuit. A heated cuvette (41°C) is incorporated to prevent water vapour condensation.

Side stream analysers sample the gases at a rate of 150–200 ml/min. There is a delay in response. The sampling tube has a 1.2 mm internal diameter and is ideally less than 2 m long.

What are the limitations of capnography?

- May not give the trend of $PaCO_2$ if there is V/Q mismatch. In patients with chronic obstructive airway disease (COAD) the waveform shows a sloping trace and does not accurately reflect $ETCO_2$.
- It is unreliable at high respiratory rates. Patient's tidal breath can be diluted with fresh gas.
- Dilution of the end tidal CO_2 can occur whenever there are loose connections and system leaks.
- Nitrous oxide absorbs infrared light with an absorption spectrum overlapping with that of CO_2. This causes inaccuracy of the detector, N_2O being interpreted as CO_2. This can be avoided by careful choice of wavelength using special filters.
- Error can occur due to collision broadening.
- Does not monitor oxygenation!

What do you mean by collision broadening?

Collision broadening is the increased absorption of CO_2 due to the presence of nitrous oxide or nitrogen.

Following absorption of the infrared rays by a CO_2 molecule there is an increase in its rotational and vibrational energy. In the presence of nitrous oxide, by colliding with those molecules, CO_2 can transfer some of its absorbed energy to nitrous oxide. Now, CO_2 can absorb more energy from infra-red beam than it would in the absence of nitrous oxide. This effect is called 'collision broadening'.

By calibrating with a gas mixture that contains the same background gases as the sample this potential error can be prevented.

Q3 Filters

Why do you use breathing system filters?

To prevent the contamination of breathing system and to prevent cross infection.

What mechanisms are involved in the filtration of micro-organisms?

- *Interception*: Particles with diameters larger than the pore size are intercepted by the fibres of the filter.
- *Inertial impaction*: Particles strike the fibres because of its inertia.
- *Diffusion*: particles less than 0.1 μm undergo Brownian motion and are captured.
- *Gravity*: Large particles settle on the fibres due to gravity.
- *Electrostatic attraction*.

Do you know any types of breathing system filters?

- *Pleated hydrophobic membrane filters*: Large membrane (contains resin-bonded ceramic fibres) is folded (pleated). The design prevents the ingress of water droplets.
- *Electrostatic or composite filters*: Hygroscopic layer and a large pore felt filter. The felt (matted fabric) is subjected to electric field to improve the filtration performance.

What is filtration performance?

Filtration performance is determined by *penetration*. Penetration is the number of particles passing through the filter as a percentage of the number of particles in the challenge to the filter.

Efficiency is (100 − penetration) % (e.g. pleated filter, for virus; penetration is 0.00014–0.0047%). Efficiency: 99.99986–99.9953%.

Can you name the factors affecting filtration efficiency?

Density of fibres and depth of filter. Increasing these will increase the efficiency, but also increase the resistance.

What is the pore size in a standard blood filter and why do you use it?

It is about 170 μm. This is to filter clots and debris.

Can this filter the micro-aggregates?

No. There are micro-aggregate filters with pore size 20–40 μm. They are of various types, depth filters, screen filters, or combination filters. Screen filters have sieves with pores. Depth filters remove particles by adsorbing them.

Can you tell some harmful effects of micro-aggregates?

- Febrile transfusion reaction
- Pulmonary injury; micro-embolic blockage of pre-capillary arterioles
- Thrombocytopaenia

What are the problems in using micro-aggregate filters?

Micro-aggregate filters are not used commonly for general purposes. The problems in using them include:

- Haemolysis
- Resistance to flow
- Platelet retention
- Adsorption of immunoglobulins
- Release of foreign particles into the blood
- Paradoxically, can trigger micro-aggregate formation in the recipient by complement activation

SOE 2

Physiology 2

Key topics: acid–base, thyroid, coronary circulation

Q1 Acid–base balance

Can you define pH?

pH is the negative logarithm to the base 10 of hydrogen ion concentration.

What is the relationship between H^+ ions and pH?

$$
\begin{aligned}
\text{pH } 7.0 &= 100\,\text{nmol/l (i.e. } 10^{-7}\,\text{mol/l)}\\
\text{pH } 8.0 &= 10\,\text{nmol/l}\\
\text{pH } 6.0 &= 1000\,\text{nmol/l}
\end{aligned}
$$

What is the Henderson–Hasselbalch equation? Can you derive it?

$$\text{pH} \propto HCO_3^-/H_2CO_3 \qquad \text{pH} = 6.1 + \log\,[HCO_3^-/H_2CO_3]$$

The law of mass action states that at equilibrium, the ratio of product/concentration of opposing reaction sets is a constant. (The law states that the rate of any given chemical reaction is proportional to the product of the concentrations of the reactants.) Therefore:

$$
\begin{aligned}
HA &\leftrightarrow H^+ + A^-\\
K &= (H^+)(A^-)/HA\\
H^+ &= K(HA)/A^-\\
\text{pH} = \text{pK} + \log A^-/HA &= 6.1 + \log\,[HCO_3^-/H_2CO_3]\\
\text{pH} &= 6.1 + \log\,[HCO_3^-/0.2 \times PCO_2\ (\text{kPa})]
\end{aligned}
$$

How is the normal acid–base balance maintained?

H^+ concentration is normally maintained within strict limits by buffering of H^+ ions and elimination of H^+ ions.

What do you mean buffering? Name some buffers and tell me how they work.

Buffering is the property of solution that resists any change in acid–base status. It typically consists of a weak acid and its salt with its conjugate base.

Buffers can broadly be classified as extracellular and intracellular.

- *Extracellular buffers*:
  - Bicarbonate
  - Haemoglobin (can also be considered as intracellular as it is within red cells)
  - Phosphate in urine
  - Calcium bicarbonate in bone.
- *Intracellular buffers*:
  - Proteins
  - Phosphates.

The effectiveness of a buffer system is determined by the pKa. The closer the pKa to the physiological pH, the more effective the system will be. The pKa of the phosphate system and that of haemoglobin is 6.8 whereas the bicarbonate buffer system has a pKa of 6.1. This means the phosphate buffer system is more efficient than bicarbonate but bicarbonate accounts for 65% of total buffering capacity. This enhanced effectiveness of the bicarbonate buffer system is because of its dual role in both kidneys and lungs.

Proteins contribute 5% of total buffering capacity and have a pKa of 7.4. Proteins have a free COOH group and free NH_3^+ group which can dissociate.

Haemoglobin is responsible for 29% of total buffering capacity, deoxyhaemoglobin being a better buffer than oxyhaemoglobin:

$$HbO_2 \rightarrow Hb + O_2$$
$$Hb + H^+ \rightarrow HHb$$

How is H^+ ion eliminated and what is the role of kidney in this regard?

- *Rapid* elimination by respiratory system.
- *Slow* elimination by renal system: Formation of dihydrogen phosphate, ammonia secretion and reabsorption of filtered bicarbonate.

What is an anion gap?

The anion gap is the difference between the measured cations and anions. $(Na^+ + K^+) - (Cl^- + HCO_3^-)$, normal value is 12–18 mmol/l.

This gap is due to unmeasured anions (proteins in the anionic form, phosphates, sulphates and organic acids).

Q2 Thyroid gland

What hormones are secreted by the thyroid gland?

Thyroxine (T_4), tri-iodothyronine (T_3) and small amounts of reverse T_3.

What are their functions?

- Calorigenic effect, which increases basal metabolic rate (BMR), increases oxygen consumption (metabolism of fatty acids, increases membrane bound $Na^+ - K^+$ ATPase in many tissues).
- Development of nervous system.
- Effect on reflexes (reaction time to stretch reflexes is shortened in hyperthyroidism).
- Sensitise myocardium to catecholamines. Thyroid hormones also have a direct effect on myocytes, increases the level of α isoform of myosin heavy chain.
- Lower plasma cholesterol.
- Potentiate the effects of growth hormone.
- Increase the rate of carbohydrate absorption.

What is the mechanism of action of thyroid hormone?

Thyroid hormone enters the cells and binds to the thyroid receptor in the nuclei. The hormone–receptor complex then binds to the DNA and alters the expression of genes that code for enzymes regulating the cell function. T_3 is more potent and acts more rapidly than T_4.

What steps are involved in the formation of thyroid hormones?

- Iodination of tyrosine (tyrosine is present in thyroglobulin).
- Iodide enters the thyroid gland via $Na^+ - K^+$ ATPase pump.
- Monoiodotyrosine is formed.
- Monoiodotyrosine combines with oxidised iodine to form diiodotyrosine.
- Condensation of two molecules of di-iodotyrosine to form T_4 under the influence of thyroid stimulating hormone (TSH).
- Condensation of monoiodotyrosine and di-iodotyrosine to form T_3.
- TSH causes release of T_3 and T_4.

Q3 Coronary circulation

What is the normal coronary blood flow?

Normal coronary blood flow is about 250 ml/min (about 5% of cardiac output (CO)).

What are the various methods that can be used to study coronary blood flow?

- Using the Fick principle. This states that the blood flow to any organ = Qx/[Ax − Vx]. Otherwise expressed as the amount of substance or tracer taken up or given off by an organ in unit time is equal to the product of the blood flow through the organ and the concentration difference of the substance across the organ. Note that inhaled nitrous oxide is used in this instance. Where:
  - Qx is the amount of substance removed by the organ;
  - Ax is the arterial concentration;
  - Vx is the venous concentration from coronary sinus (requires catheterisation of coronary sinus).
- Thermodilution techniques.
- Radionuclide scanning (thallium scan).
- Coronary angiography (to assess regional blood flow).

Can you draw me a diagram representing left and right coronary artery blood flow over time (i.e. during ventricular systole and diastole)?

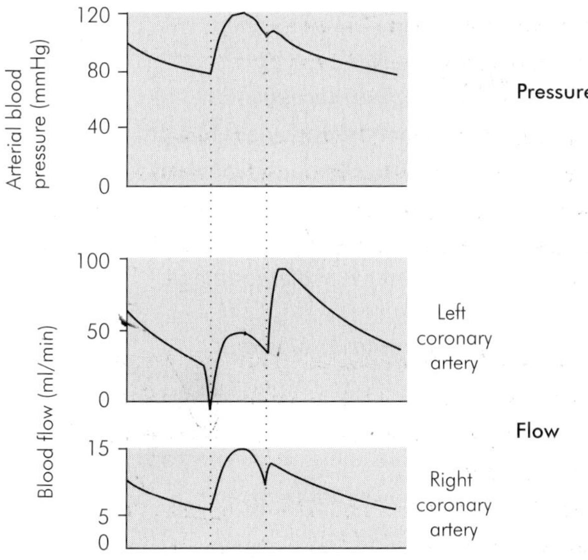

Figure 2.1 *Coronary blood flow and the cardiac cycle*

What is the significance of subendocardial blood supply?

Blood flow to the subendocardium of the *left ventricle* occurs during diastole (perfusion pressure of about 75 mmHg). During systole this perfusion pressure to the left ventricle falls to 0 mmHg. The intraventricular pressure increases during systole compressing the subendocardial vessels which ceases the blood flow.

What factors affect coronary blood flow?

Flow = pressure/resistance ($Q = P/R$). Therefore, flow will be affected by the coronary perfusion pressure (which is aortic diastolic pressure – left ventricular end-diastolic pressure) and the various factors (neural, hormonal and extravascular mechanical compression) that affect the resistance of coronary vasculature:

- *Heart rate*: Tachycardia reduces diastolic time and reduces blood flow.
- *Chemical factors*: such as vasodilator metabolites; CO_2, H^+, K^+, lactate, prostaglandins and adenosine. This is determined by the metabolic demand.
- *Neural factors*: Vagal stimulation causes coronary dilation. Alpha-adrenergic stimulation causes vasoconstriction, beta-adrenergic stimulation causes vasodilation.

Pharmacology 2

Key topics: pharmacokinetics, local anaesthetic agents, anticoagulants

Q1 Pharmacokinetics

What do you mean by the term pharmacokinetics?

Pharmacokinetics describes what the body does to a drug. It concerns the absorption, distribution, metabolism and elimination of drugs.

Which drugs can be administered by a transdermal route?

Glyceryl trinitrate, hyoscine, fentanyl, ethinylestradiol.

What factors influence transdermal absorption?

The lipid lamellar bilayers of stratum corneum prevent the penetration of polar compounds. Some potent drugs with high lipid solubility may still be absorbed transdermally. In these conditions the stratum corneum may act as a reservoir for these drugs. The absorption can be increased by the use of various penetration enhancers.

The contact surface area of the patch with the skin and concentration of the drug administered are the other important factors.

What are the advantages of transdermal route?

- Avoids first-pass effect.
- Slow and sustained absorption.
- Steady plasma level without significant troughs and peaks.
- Can be useful when enteral route is not tolerated.

What is bioavailability?

Bioavailability is the fraction of the administered dose that reaches the systemic circulation. Bioavailability is 100% for intravenous injection. It varies from 0% to 100% for other routes depending on absorption, first-pass hepatic metabolism, etc.

What factors affect bioavailability?

- *Route of administration.*
- *Pharmaceutical preparations*: particle size, presence of binding agents preventing drug dissolution, ionisation state, lipid and water solubility, protein binding.
- *Interactions*: presence of other drugs, food, induction of hepatic enzymes.
- *Patient factors*: congenital or acquired mal-absorption syndromes, coeliac disease, sprue.
- *Organ perfusion.*
- *First-pass metabolism.*

What do you mean by 'first-pass metabolism'?

After oral administration, removal of the absorbed drugs from the hepatic sinusoids and metabolism before the drug reaches the systemic circulation is called first-pass metabolism. First-pass metabolism by the liver is common with drugs that have high hepatic extraction ratio. Examples are: propranolol, opioid and lidocaine.

How may bioavailability be measured?

Bioavailability can be measured by plotting the graph of plasma concentration (C_p) against time for the test route and intravenous dose and then finding the ratio (F) of the area under the respective curves.

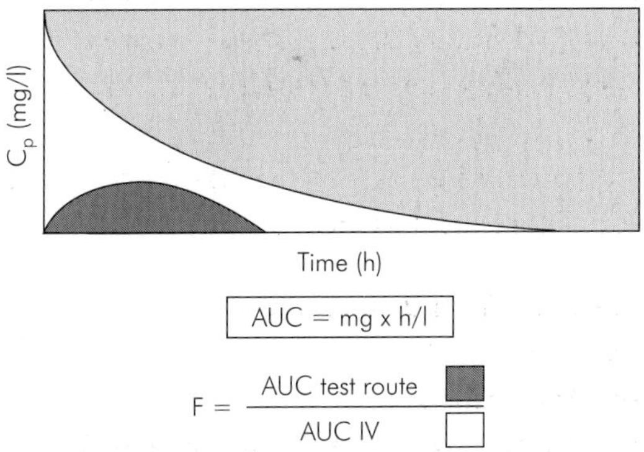

Figure 2.2 *Bioavailability*

Q2 Local anaesthetic agents

What sort of drugs are local anaesthetics?

Local anaesthetics are drugs that can reversibly block nerve conduction. They have a membrane stabilising effect due to blockade of sodium channels.

Can you classify local anaesthetics?

They can be amides or esters depending upon the chemical link between the amino and aromatic chain.

Compare and contrast amide and ester local anaesthetics.

Table 2.1 *Amide and ester local anaesthetics*

Property	Amide	Ester
Link	CO–NH	O = C – O
Stability	Stable	Relatively unstable
Metabolism	Amidases in liver	Esterases in blood
Hypersensitive reactions	Very rare	Due to *p*-amino Benzoic acid
Example	Lidocaine, bupivacaine	Cocaine, procaine

Tell me how local-anaesthetic drugs act.

Most local anaesthetics are weak bases. When deposited in tissues (which normally have alkaline pH) they dissociate into ionised and unionised forms. The unionised form can cross the biological membranes and enter into the neurons. Within the nerve cell the molecules again dissociate into ionised and unionised form. Here the ionised component blocks the sodium channels from inside and blocks the conduction of impulses.

What physical properties of these drugs affect onset, potency and duration of block?

- *Onset*: pKa.
- *Potency*: lipid solubility.
- *Duration*: amount of drug, lipid solubility and protein binding.

What do you mean by pKa? What is its significance?

pKa is the negative logarithm of the dissociation constant (K). This is the pH in which the given drug equally dissociates into its ionised and unionised form. The closer the pKa to the physiological pH, the faster will be the onset of drug.

Can you compare bupivacaine and lidocaine?

Table 2.2 *Bupivacaine and lidocaine*

Property	Bupivacaine	Lidocaine
Chemical nature	Amide	Amide
pKa	8.1	7.8
Lipid solubility	++++	+
Protein binding	96%	64%
Onset of action	Moderate	Faster
Duration of action	Longer (2–8 h)	Shorter (1–2 h)
Potency	++++(×4 times)	+
Toxicity	Cardiotoxicity +++	+
Dose	2 mg/kg	3 mg/kg (7 mg/kg with epinephrine)

How does levobupivacaine differ from bupivacaine?

Bupivacaine is a racemic mixture. Levobupivacaine is the levorotatory enantiomer of racemic bupivacaine. Clinically it is similar to normal bupivacaine. The important difference claimed based on animal studies is lower cardiotoxicity. The maximum recommended dose remains the same at 2 mg/kg.

What are the advantages of ropivacaine over bupivacaine?

Ropivacaine, like bupivacaine, is an amide local anaesthetic. It is less lipid soluble than bupivacaine and hence its penetration in neuronal myelin sheath is limited. C fibres which are thin and unmyelinated are blocked more readily than the thick and well myelinated A fibres. Therefore, at lower concentrations the sensory blockade is more than motor. In higher-concentration motor blockade is similar to bupivacaine. This sparing of the motor blockade at lower concentrations is the main advantage of ropivacaine over bupivacaine. The cardiotoxicity of ropivacaine is also less than that of bupivacaine.

What is EMLA cream?

EMLA stands for eutectic mixture of local anaesthetics. It is a mixture of 2.5% prilocaine and 2.5% lidocaine used for topical anaesthesia.

What do you mean by a eutectic mixture?

A eutectic mixture is one in which the constituents are in such proportions that the freezing (or melting) point is as low as possible, with the constituents freezing (or melting) simultaneously.

Q3 Anticoagulants

What are the anticoagulants commonly used in clinical practice?

The two main types of anticoagulants used in clinical practice include heparin and vitamin K antagonists (e.g. warfarin).

Can you describe the structure of heparin?

Heparin is a naturally occurring negatively charged acid. It is a glycosaminoglycan formed from alternating residues of L-iduronic acid and D-glucosamine. It has a complex sulphated polysaccharide structure. The molecular weight of unfractionated heparin (UFH) ranges widely from 3000 to 30,000 Da with an average of about 15,000 Da.

Tell me about the mechanism of action of heparin.

Heparin acts indirectly via the α_2-globulin called antithrombin III. Antithrombin III in turn activates serine proteases of the coagulation cascade thereby exerting an inhibitory effect on the cascade. Although antithrombin III normally has a low level of intrinsic activity, in the presence of heparin, the reaction with thrombin increases several thousand fold.

In low-doses heparin binds to antithrombin III accelerating its combination with thrombin to form an inactive complex. Activated factor Xa is inhibited by a similar mechanism. At higher C_p activated factors IXa, XIa and XIIa are also inhibited. Heparin also reduces platelet aggregation at higher doses.

What is low molecular weight heparin (LMWH)?

LMWH are products of chemical or enzymatic depolymerisation of UFH. Unlike UFH, LMWH have molecular weights of 4000–6500 Da. There are various commercial preparations available (e.g. enoxaparin, dalteparin).

Can you list the differences between UFH and LMWH?

1 LMWH are 2–3 times more potent in factor Xa inhibition when compared to UFH.
2 In contrast to UFH which is more than 50% protein bound only 10% of LMWH is bound to protein.
3 Following subcutaneous administration LMWH is not as rapidly degraded as UFH. UFH has a bioavailability of 40% whereas absorption is more complete with LMWH.
4 The half-life of UFH is dose dependent varying from 30 min (with a dose of 25 units/kg) to 150 min (with a dose of 400 units/kg). The half-life of LMWH is 2–4 times as long as UFH with corresponding doses.
5 The higher bioavailability and longer half-life allow once daily subcutaneous administration of LMWH. The anticoagulant response is more predictable.

6 UFH is monitored with activated partial thromboplastin time (APTT). Although the activity of LMWH is usually not monitored, an anti-Xa assay is available to monitor the effect, especially in high-risk patients.

How can you reverse the action of heparin?

UFH has a relatively shorter half-life and if the clinical situation permits one can wait for the effect to wear off. Alternatively protamine can be used. This is extracted from fish sperm and is very strongly basic. It combines with the strong acid, heparin to form stable inactive complex.

How does warfarin work?

Warfarin acts by antagonising vitamin K. Vitamin K is necessary for the carboxylation of glutamate residues of factors II, VII, IX and X. This carboxylation is coupled to the conversion of vitamin K from the reduced to the oxidised form. This is impaired by warfarin.

Oral anticoagulants inhibit the enzyme epoxide reductase and cofactor nicotinamide adenine dinucleotide (NADH) which are responsible for regeneration of the reduced form of vitamin K, thereby preventing the activation of the above factors.

How long will it take for warfarin to exert its effect and how will you monitor it?

Following oral administration the peak plasma concentration occurs in about 90 min but it will take about 3 days of daily dosing to achieve a steady state concentration. The half-life of warfarin is about 36 h. Although the clinical effect is apparent in 8–24 h following ingestion of warfarin, it takes 3–5 days to reach the desired therapeutic effect.

The effect of warfarin is monitored by prothrombin time (PT) or the international normalised ratio (INR).

Tell me about drug interaction with warfarin?

Warfarin in about 97% protein bound. It is metabolised in liver and excreted in kidney, so there can be a significant degree of interaction with various drugs.

- Interactions increasing the effect of warfarin:
  - Competition for protein binding sites (e.g. non-steroidal anti-inflammatory drugs (NSAIDs) and diuretics).
  - Increased hepatic binding (e.g. T_4).
  - Inhibition of hepatic microsomal enzymes.
  - Reduced vitamin K synthesis (e.g. broad spectrum antibiotics – by reducing gut flora).
  - Synergistic anti-haemostatic actions (e.g. antiplatelet drugs-aspirin, clopidogrel).

- Interactions decreasing the effect of warfarin:
  - Induction of hepatic microsomal enzymes (e.g. phenytoin).
  - Increased level of clotting factors (e.g. oestrogen – increase level of vitamin K dependent factors).
  - Binding of warfarin in gut (e.g. cholestyramine).
  - Increased vitamin K intake.

How can you reverse the effect of warfarin?

This depends on the clinical situation and the urgency and is often done after discussing with the haematologists.

With normal liver function a dose of vitamin K can reverse the effect of warfarin in 4–6 h. This can increase the risks of thromboembolism as it takes up to a week to re-establish the anticoagulant effect of warfarin following vitamin K administration.

More commonly fresh frozen plasma (FFP) in a dose of 10–15 ml/kg reverses the effect of warfarin transiently.

Clinical 2

Key topics: intravenous drug abuse, smoking, local anaesthetic toxicity

Q1 A 38-year-old male – an intravenous drug abuser in the past and a heavy smoker is on the emergency list for incision and drainage of abscess on the anterior aspect of his thigh.

Can you summarise the problems encountered in anaesthetising this patient?

The problems encountered are secondary to the history of drug abuse, smoking and the need for urgent surgery with limited time for preparation.

What are the challenges in managing an intravenous drug abuser?

- Poor historians.
- May be drowsy or agitated and uncooperative.
- Coexisting infective disease is common.
- Difficult venous access.
- Altered response to anaesthetic drugs.
- Theatre contamination.
- High requirements for post-operative pain relief.

What hazards of smoking are you worried about?

- *Respiratory system*: Irritable airway, copious secretions, impaired tracheobronchial clearance, small airway narrowing, higher closing capacity (exceeds FRC), atelectasis, and coexisting chronic obstructive airway disease (COAD). Heavy smokers have a greater tendency to develop post-operative hypoxia and chest infection.
- *Cardiovascular system*: Nicotine increases heart rate, blood pressure and produces vasoconstriction. Smokers have increased blood viscosity and develop polycythaemia. Smoking increases the level of carboxyhaemoglobin which reduces oxygen delivery. Coexisting ischaemic heart disease and peripheral vascular disease are common.
- *Immune function*: Decreased levels of immunoglobulins and white cells. Due to adverse effects on microcirculation, wound healing can be delayed.

What are the benefits of stopping smoking pre-operatively? How long prior to surgery do smokers need to give up smoking to get these benefits?

As the half-life of carboxyhaemoglobin is 4 h, stopping smoking for 4–12 h improves the oxygen delivery.

Within 12–24 h the effect of nicotine systemically is greatly reduced.

At 6–8 weeks ciliary activity is restored and sputum production declines. Immunological function returns to normal after 6 months.

What options are available to manage difficult venous access?

- Inhalational induction. This should be discussed with the patient during pre-operative assessment.
- External jugular vein cannulation.
- Femoral vein cannulation.
- Internal jugular vein cannulation.
- Ultrasound guidance should be used for cannulating major veins.

What precautions will you take to anaesthetise this patient?

Precautions should be taken to provide personal safety, staff safety and patient safety.

Universal precautions should be strictly followed. Appropriate communication with other theatre staff is essential. Anaesthetising the patient in theatre rather than anaesthetic room minimises contamination. All sharps should be disposed of safely. Single use breathing equipments should be used where possible. Any reusable equipment should be sterilised immediately after the use.

What do you mean by universal precautions? How will you protect yourself?

Universal precautions are infection control guidelines designed to protect workers from exposure. All patients should be assumed to be infectious for blood-borne diseases such as human immunodeficiency virus (HIV) and hepatitis B (diseases spread by blood and certain body fluids).

What will you do if you sustain an accidental needle stick injury to your finger?
Encourage free bleeding by squeezing the finger. Wash hands thoroughly with soap and water. Report the accident to the department manager and seek advice from occupational health department.

Arrange personal test for hepatitis B antibody titre. After obtaining consent from the patient, collect patient blood sample for hepatitis B/HIV.

Passive immunisation with hepatitis B immunoglobulin, antiviral drugs, antibiotics, antitetanus immunisation should be considered.

Can you name some antiviral drugs?
These are mainly classified into two groups:
- *Nucleoside reverse transcriptase inhibitors*: zidovudine, stavudine.
- *Protease inhibitors*: amprenavir, ritonavir.

How will you anaesthetise this patient?
Complete pre-operative assessment, communication with the surgeon and theatre staff. Likely choice either spinal anaesthetic or general anaesthetic with femoral nerve block.

What are the benefits of spinal anaesthetic in this patient?
As this is a short surgical procedure, spinal anaesthesia extends to the post-operative period and provides immediate post-operative analgesia. The use of anaesthetic breathing circuits and ancillary equipment can be avoided.

In addition there are other benefits of spinal anaesthesia such as minimal effect on respiratory function, reduced incidence of deep vein thrombosis etc. (further details in SOE 10).

How will you manage his post-operative pain relief?
Regular medication that the patient may have been receiving such as methadone, should be continued.

Analgesics with opioid-sparing effects – paracetamol and NSAIDs.
- *Regional analgesia*: Femoral nerve block.
- *Opioids*: Oral morphine preparation (oramorph).

You have planned general anaesthesia and femoral nerve block for this patient. You decide to do the nerve block awake.

Describe how you will perform a femoral nerve block.

1 Preparation of patient: includes explanation of the technique, benefits and complications. Obtain consent.
2 Preparation of theatre: includes having a trained assistant for help, checking the equipment – both for performance of the block (nerve stimulator, regional block needle) and for resuscitation (airway equipment, anaesthetic machine check).
3 Secure intravenous access and establish monitoring.
4 Preparation of site: includes positioning the patient and aseptic precautions; identify the anatomical land marks: inguinal ligament, femoral artery.
5 Performance of block: 50 mm long insulated nerve stimulator needle is used. Needle is inserted 1 cm below the inguinal ligament and 1 cm lateral to the femoral artery at about 45° to the skin and slowly advanced using nerve stimulator, observing for patellar twitches. 20–30 ml of local anaesthetic is injected in small aliquots after careful negative aspiration. Failure of the twitches to disappear either with very low stimulation current or after starting injection of local anaesthetic and undue resistance or shooting pain during injection may infer intraneural injection.

Which local anaesthetic drugs can be used?

Lidocaine 1%, prilocaine 1%, levobupivacaine 0.25–0.5% or bupivacaine 0.25–0.5%.

Q2 Critical incident: local anaesthetic toxicity

As you inject about 20 ml of 0.375% bupivacaine patient mentions that he feels light headed and has tingling around his lips and tongue.

What are you going to do?

- Recognise this as a possible intravascular injection of bupivacaine.
- Stop injecting.
- Call for help, reassure patient.

As you are watching he starts fitting. What will you do?

- Assess and manage Airway, Breathing and Circulation. Give 100% Oxygen.
- Check pulse, blood pressure, oxygen saturation and electrocardiogram (ECG).
- Diazepam 2.5 mg, lorazepam 4 mg or thiopental 50 mg intravenously.

His blood pressure is 60/30 mmHg and heart rate 38/min; he stops breathing.

Secure his airway with tracheal intubation and ventilate with 100% oxygen. Intravenous fluids (colloid or crystalloid), ephedrine 6 mg, atropine 0.3–0.6 mg intravenously.

In spite of all your attempts he becomes persistently bradycardic and his ECG shows this rhythm. How will you proceed?

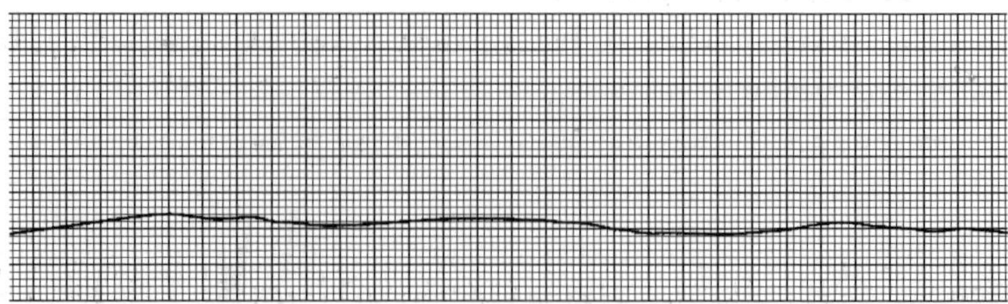

Figure 2.3 *Rhythm strip: asystole*

- Check pulse.
- If no pulse, follow ALS algorithm.
- CPR for 3 min with each loop of algorithm, assess ECG rhythm.
- Epinephrine 1 mg intravenous every 3 min.
- Atropine 3 mg intravenous once only.
- External pacing if there are any p waves or slow ventricular activity on the ECG.

Q3 What are the factors affecting local anaesthetic toxicity?

CVS and central nervous system (CNS) effects depend on the total amount of drug reaching the systemic circulation. This is influenced by following factors:

- Total dose of drug administered.
- Site of injection (intercostals > epidural > plexus > peripheral nerve block > subcutaneous).
- Tissue protein binding and metabolism.
- Vascularity of the injection site.

What physiological systems are affected by local anaesthetic toxicity?
The two major systems which are affected are the CNS and CVS. The effect on the neurological system is said to be biphasic. The inhibitory neurons are affected first and this leads to a general increase in activity with agitation followed by grand mal-type convulsions. Secondarily there is a general depression of all nervous system activity with unconsciousness, cardiovascular depression and apnoea.

The cadiovascular centres in the brain are depressed and the effect of local anaesthetic agents on the heart is a broadening of the QRS complex often associated with brady arrhythmias and hypotension.

The effects of local-anaesthetic agents are due to their effects on the sodium channel and effectively a general membrane stabilising effect.

What precautions should you take to avoid local anaesthetic toxicity?

- Total dose of local anaesthetic should be carefully calculated. Keep within maximum recommended dose guidelines.
- Safest drug available should be chosen (when possible, e.g. levobupivacaine instead of bupivacaine).
- Inject very slowly and aspirate at every 4–5 ml of injection.

Physics, clinical measurement and safety 2

Key topics: neuromuscular monitoring, blood pressure, endotracheal tubes

Q1 Monitoring of neuromuscular function

Why should we monitor neuromuscular function?

Monitoring helps in the delivery of the appropriate dose of relaxant, helps to detect the type of block, monitor the depth of block and helps assess adequate recovery.

Relying on standard pharmacokinetic data in dosing muscle relaxants is unreliable owing to great patient-to-patient variability.

How can neuromuscular function be monitored?

Monitoring can be based on clinical parameters or by using neuromuscular stimulation equipment.

The clinical parameters include:

- Grip strength.
- Ability to sustain head lift for at least 5 s.
- Ability to produce vital capacity of at least 10 ml/kg.

Note: Measurement of tidal volume does not provide a reliable guide to adequacy of reversal. A normal tidal volume can be achieved with only 20% return of diaphragmatic power. As these measurements are not possible in an anaesthetised patient, a more commonly employed method is use of a peripheral nerve stimulator.

What are the common methods of measuring the response of the muscle to stimulation?

- *Transcutaneous electrical stimulation (TCES)*: A TCE stimulation is given near a nerve and the response assessed with vision and touch.
- *Mechanomyography*: This uses a force transducer to quantitatively measure contractile response.

- *Acceleromyography*: Muscle movement causing movement of joint is measured.
- *Electromyography*: Measures electrical activity associated with the propagation of action potential in muscle cells. Not widely used clinically.

Which nerves can be used for stimulation?

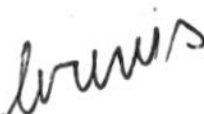

- Most commonly used is ulnar nerve (adductor pollicis – adducts thumb).
- Zygomatic branch of facial nerve – orbicularis oculi muscle.
- Peroneal nerve/post-tibial nerve – dorsiflexion of foot and plantar flexion of big toe.

Where will you place the stimulating electrode?

Negative – black coloured – generates action potential by depolarising the membrane. Depolarisation (versus hyperpolarisation by the positive electrode) makes it easier to stimulate the nerve. Maximum twitch height occurs when negative electrode is placed in closest proximity to the nerve (***N***egative on the ***N***erve).

Discuss important characteristics of the peripheral nerve stimulator?

Portable, battery powered. Should be able to deliver impulses of:

- 0.3 ms duration to prevent repetitive firing of the nerve.
- Supramaximal current output of 50–60 mA at all frequencies – guarantees that all nerve fibres depolarises.
- Monophasic square wave pulse waveform – constant current for a specified interval.
- Single twitch at 0.1 Hz, Train of four (TOF) at 2 Hz, Tetanic stimulation at 50 Hz.

What are the characteristic responses to the various patterns of stimulation produced by non-depolarising (NDMR) and depolarising (DMR) agents?

- *NDMR*: Repetitive stimulation (TOF or tetanus) is associated with fade and post-tetanic facilitation.
- *DMR*: No fade or post-tetanic facilitation (but Phase II block with suxamethonium can give characteristics of NDMR).

What is the TOF?

'TOF' is a mode of stimulation at 2 Hz to estimate the degree of block.

Four stimuli are given at 0.5 s intervals. TOF is more sensitive than single twitches in monitoring neuromuscular blockade.

It is described as the ratio of the force generated by the fourth contraction compared with the force at the first contraction ($T_4:T_1$).

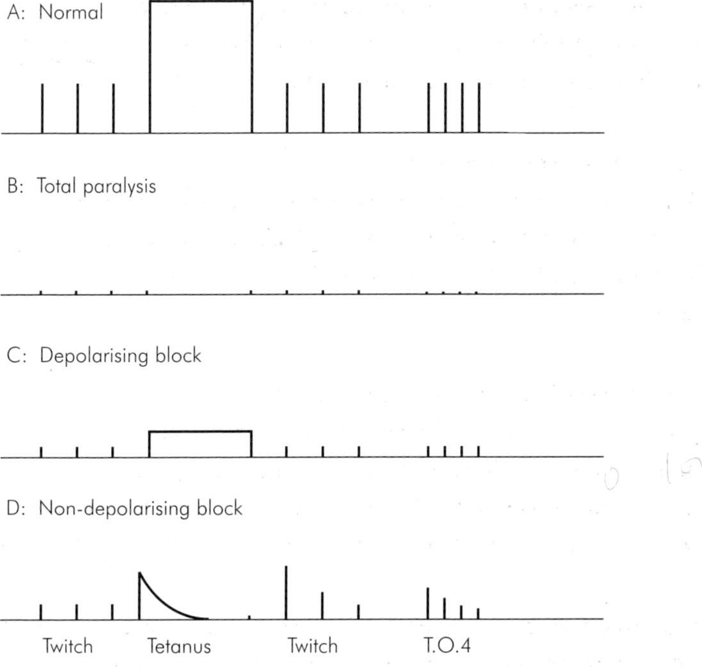

Figure 2.4 *Responses for single twitch and TOF*

As transducers are not generally used in day-to-day practice, monitoring TOF count is more clinically relevant.

TOF count	Extent of block
1,2,3	75% (T_4 is lost)
1,2	80% (T_4, T_3 lost)
1	90% (T_4, T_3, T_2 lost)
0	100% (T_4, T_3, T_2, T_1 lost)

What is double-burst stimulation?

This is a relatively recent introduction in neuromuscular monitoring in which manual assessment of fade is made more reliable. Two bursts of tetanic stimulation at 50 Hz, separated by 750 ms, are given. Each burst is further made up of three tetanic twitches at 20 ms intervals. Twitches T_1 and T_2 are clinically detected. The $T_2 : T_1$ ratio depends on the degree of block. This is similar to TOF ratio but tactile evaluation is more sensitive with this pattern.

Q2 Measurement of blood pressure

What are the methods available for measuring blood pressure?

Blood pressure can be measured by non-invasive indirect methods and invasive direct methods. The non-invasive methods include:

- Manometer (mercury and aneroid).
- von Recklinghausen oscillotonometer.
- Automated oscillometric technique.
- Penaz technique (Finapres).
- Microphone/Doppler.

Who was Korotkoff and what are the different phases of Korotkoff's sound?

Korotkoff was a Russian physician. The sound he described has 5 phases: Phase I begins with the appearance of sounds and corresponds to systolic pressure; Phase II is slight muffling; in Phase III there is a rise in volume; Phase IV is a fall in the sound level and Phase V is total disappearance of sounds. Phase V is accepted as diastolic pressure.

Tell me about the von Recklinghausen oscillotonometer.

This device uses double cuff. The proximal cuff is for measuring pressure and is attached to measuring bellows. The distal cuff is for detecting pulsations and is connected to another bellow. The needle in the aneroid gauge will start oscillating when systolic pressure is reached. The maximum oscillation occurs at mean blood pressure.

What is the principle behind automated non-invasive devices (DINAMAP type)?

Similar in design to the von Recklinghausen oscillotonometer, but uses a single cuff and instead of bellows a pressure transducer measures the pressure and oscillations. Microprocessor controls the inflation, deflation and display of numerical value.

For the first reading the cuff is inflated to a suitable high value (around 160 mmHg), during subsequent reading, cuff is inflated to a value about 25 mmHg above the previous reading. Cuff is deflated by 2–3 mmHg/s.

What are the disadvantages of non-invasive techniques?

- Erroneous readings with inappropriate cuff size.
- Inaccurate in the presence of arrhythmias.
- Cannot use less than 1 min interval.
- Not reliable in extremes of blood pressure (underestimates when too high and vice versa).

- Pressure effects when used for prolonged time and frequent reading resulting in petechiae, nerve palsy.

What are the indications for direct arterial blood pressure measurement?

- Cases where rapid blood pressure changes is anticipated as in cardiovascular instability, major blood loss, fluid shifts, intracranial surgery, induced hypotension.
- Need for frequent arterial blood gas analysis.
- Cases where non-invasive blood pressure may be inaccurate: arrhythmias, morbidly obese patient.

What are the problems associated with direct arterial monitoring?

Due to cannula:

- Arterial obstruction-distal ischaemia due to thrombus, haematoma.
- Bleeding.
- Infection.

Due to transducing system:

- Resonance.
- Damping.

What information can be obtained from an arterial waveform?

Rate, rhythm, myocardial contractility (slope of upstroke), hypovolaemia, peripheral resistance (slope of downstroke), index of stroke volume (area under the curve up to dicrotic notch).

What does a transducer do?

Transducers convert one form of energy to another. Here it converts mechanical energy into electrical energy. Arterial pressure transducers are based on the principle of strain gauge. Stretching a wire or silicon crystal changes its electrical resistance. Arterial pressure waves move the diaphragm and alters the tension of the wire. This results in change in resistance which is measured using a Wheatstone bridge circuit.

What is natural frequency?

It is the frequency at which the system would oscillate when disturbed. It is also called 'resonant frequency'.

What factors affect natural frequency in invasive monitoring?

Natural frequency is directly proportional to the diameter of the catheter lumen. It is inversely proportional to the square root of the length of the tubing, square root of the system compliance and to the density of the fluid.

What do you mean by resonance and damping?

Resonance is the natural tendency to oscillate and damping is the tendency to resist oscillation.

What do you mean by a damped trace?

Smoothed out trace where sharp changes are not displayed – transmission of blood pressure from the artery to the transducer diaphragm is restricted. This can be due to a clot or air bubble in the tubing.

What is the problem with underdamping or overdamping?

- *Underdamping*: overestimates systolic blood pressure, underestimates diastolic blood pressure.
- *Overdamping*: underestimates systolic blood pressure, overestimates diastolic blood pressure.

Either way, the mean arterial pressure is unaffected.

How do you check for optimal damping?

By applying high-pressure flush (300 mmHg). Under-damped system oscillates for 3–4 cycles before settling at zero. Over-damped system settles to zero without any oscillations.

Optimum damping: should settle within 2–3 cycles.

What precautions you would take to avoid damping?

- Connecting tubing should be sufficiently stiff with an internal diameter 1.5–3 mm.
- The maximum length should not exceed 120 cm.
- Line should be free of bubbles, kinks, clots.
- Maintain continuous flush (4 ml/h) in the system.

Q3 Endotracheal tubes

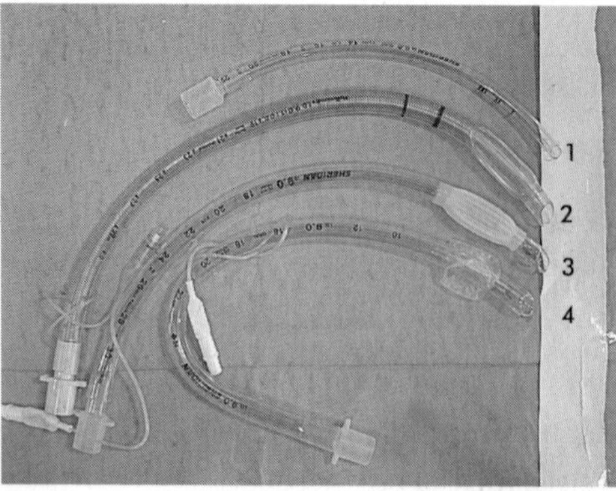

Figure 2.5 *Endotracheal tubes*

Gives picture to candidate. Identify: uncuffed (1) and cuffed (3) orotracheal tubes, armoured tracheal tube (2), RAE tube (4).

Tell me about uncuffed tubes.

Uncuffed tubes are used in children. The trauma on the delicate mucosa due to the cuff is avoided. In adults the vocal cords are the narrowest part of the airway. In the paediatric population the cricoid region is the narrowest part and is circular in cross-section and conical. If an uncuffed tube is used, of an appropriate size, it snugly fits in the sub-glottic region to provide a good seal.

How will you choose the right size and length of endotracheal tubes in children?

Size = (Age/4 + 4), length = (Age/2 + 12) for oral and (Age/2 + 15) for nasal.

What does RAE stand for?

Ring, Adair and Elwyn.

What types of endotracheal tube cuffs are you aware of?

Low pressure–high volume and low volume–high pressure cuffs.

What is the advantage of a low pressure–high volume cuff?

Pressure exerted by the cuff should be less than the mucosal perfusion pressure. In these cuffs the pressure is distributed over a larger area and hence there is a lower risk of mucosal ischaemia.

Are there any problems with the use of cuffs?

Herniation of cuff causing airway obstruction, failure to deflate at extubation and there is a theoretical risk of expansion of cuff volume when used with nitrous oxide. Prolonged use can lead to mucosal ischaemia, tracheomalacia etc.

What you know about the standardisation of endotracheal tubes?

British standard BS 3487/5 = ISO 5361.1.

This specifies that the material used in manufacturing endotracheal tubes should be resistant to deterioration in use, should be thin walled, flexible and soft whilst in use.

For the cuff: BS 3487/5 specifies a test to avoid cuff herniation. 100 g of weight on the cuff for 24 h at 40°C should fail to produce cuff herniation.

What material is used in these tubes? Why is it printed 'IT' on the tubes?

Modern day tubes are made up of polyvinyl chloride. Previously it was red rubber. 'IT' stands for 'Implantation Tested' in animals.

Do you know any other types of endotracheal tubes?

- Nasal tubes, armoured tracheal tubes.
- North and south facing RAE tubes.
- Microlaryngeal tubes.
- Flexible aluminium shaft (Mallinckrodt laserflex) or stainless steel shaft laser tubes.
- Double lumen tubes.

SOE 3

Physiology 3

Key topics: cerebral circulation, muscle, lung volumes, functional residual capacity

Q1 Cerebral circulation

What is normal cerebral blood flow (CBF)?

The normal CBF is about 50 ml/100 g/min, (grey matter: 80 ml/100 g/min, white matter: 20 ml/100 g/min). This totals about 750 ml/min which is 15% of the cardiac output (CO).

How is CBF regulated?

Flow = Pressure/resistance (Q = P/R). Therefore, CBF is proportional to the cerebral perfusion pressure (CPP) and is inversely proportional to the resistance in the cerebral vasculature.

CPP is the difference between the mean arterial pressure (MAP) and the central venous pressure (CVP) (if the intracranial pressure (ICP) is more than CVP, then CPP = MAP − ICP).

The resistance in the cerebral vasculature can be influenced by:

- Autoregulation (metabolic, pressure).
- PO_2 and PCO_2.
- Neural control.

Can you tell me more about the neural control of the cerebral circulation?

Cerebral vessels derive their sympathetic supply from the superior cervical ganglia that accompany the internal carotid artery and parasympathetic supply from facial nerve. Although the direct effect of these nerve supplies on the cerebral circulation is minimal, by altering the CO and the peripheral vascular resistance the nervous system can maintain the cerebral perfusion pressure and hence influence the CBF.

Draw me a graph indicating CBF versus $PaCO_2$ and CBF versus PaO_2? Explain the relationship in detail.

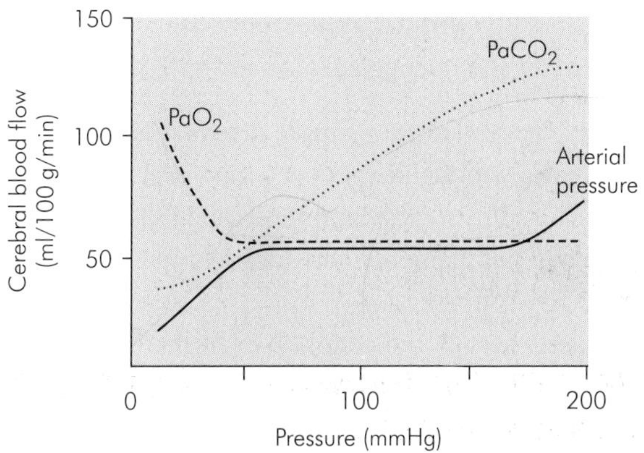

Figure 3.1 *Autoregulation of CBF*

Owing to the vasodilatory effect of carbon dioxide (CO_2) in a range of 4 kPa to about 11 kPa, there is a corresponding increase in the CBF making the relation a linear one. In contrast, PaO_2 has little effect on the CBF until less than 6.7 kPa. Below this level the CBF increases. The reason for this relationship lies in the shape of the oxygen dissociation curve. Initially, although there is a drop in the PaO_2 the oxygen content is not affected much and hence the CBF is unaltered.

How do you measure CBF?

- Kety–Schmidt technique applying the Fick principle using inhaled nitrous oxide.
- Positron emission tomography (PET), identification of differences in regional blood flow using injection of radioactive xenon.
- Doppler probes for regional flow.

Describe the Monro–Kellie doctrine.

The skull is a rigid box and ICP is a function of blood flow, amount of brain tissue and oedema, and the volume of cerebrospinal fluid within.

Can you draw a cerebral auto-regulation curve? What happens to this curve in hypertensive patients?

CBF is constant over a wide range of MAP. This curve shifts to the right in hypertensive patients. See Figure 3.1.

Q2 Muscle physiology

What different types of muscle fibres are you aware of?

Skeletal muscle, smooth muscle and cardiac muscle.

What are the functions of skeletal muscle?

- Mechanical response.
- Store for glucose and glycogen (on a short-term basis).
- Reserve for protein for gluconeogenesis (on a longer-term basis).

What is a sarcomere? Can you draw a simple structure of it?

Sarcomeres are the basic contractile units of a myofibril. Each muscle cell is made up of a myofibril enclosed by a cell membrane called sarcolemma. The myofibrils are made up of two types of filaments, the thick filament myosin and the thin filament actin.

The myosin filaments occupy the central part of the myofibril and interdigitate with actin filaments. The A-band represents the myosin filaments. The M-line is in the middle of A-band where the myosin filaments are aligned side by side. The thin actin filaments overlap the myosin and are joined at their end in the Z-line. Therefore, a sarcomere is the unit that exists between the two Z-lines. In the relaxed state, the area of myosin filaments not overlapped by the actin filaments is known as the H-zone.

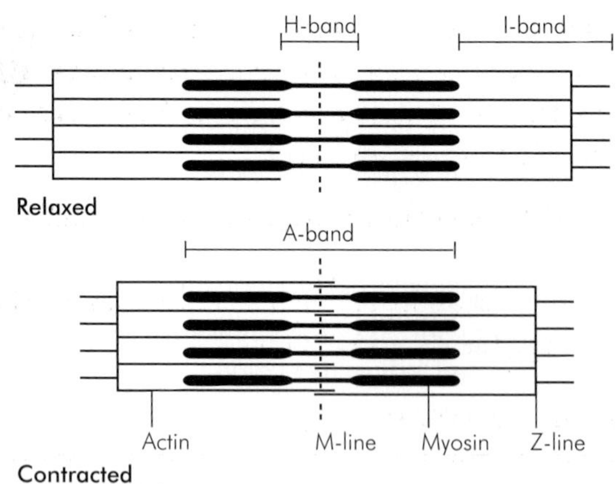

Figure 3.2 *Structure of sarcomere*

What do you understand by 'excitation–contraction coupling'?

Excitation–contraction coupling describes a cyclical event that follows excitation of a muscle that ultimately leads to contraction. Contraction of a sarcomere is caused by an interaction between actin and myosin. This involves consumption of energy provided by adenosine triphosphate (ATP) and requires calcium.

The event begins with depolarisation of sarcolemma by a nerve stimulus. This wave of depolarisation spreads along the muscle membrane and also into the depth of the muscle fibres. In the resting state, calcium is stored in the sarcoplasmic reticulum within the cells. As this depolarisation wave reaches the sarcoplasmic reticulum (along the T-tubules), calcium is released from the sarcoplasmic reticulum into themyoplasm through certain calcium release channels (also known as ryanodine receptors).

The released calcium attaches to the troponin which causes conformational changes resulting in revealing of active sites on the actin filament to which myosin can attach. Eventually there is movement between the filaments often described as 'powerstroke' that leads to contraction of muscle.

Finally relaxation occurs when there is reuptake of calcium back into the sarcoplasmic reticulum.

What is the source of energy for the muscle metabolism?

There are three different pathways that lead to formation of ATP, which is the source of energy for muscle metabolism:

- Oxidative phosphorylation.
- Glycolytic phosphorylation.
- Phosphorylation of ADP by creatine phosphate.

Of the three pathways, oxidative phosphorylation supplies most of the ATP requirements and as its name implies, needs oxygen. This process takes place in the mitochondria. In contrast, glycolytic phosphorylation takes place in the cytoplasm and does not require oxygen. Glycolytic phosphorylation is less efficient in that it produces less molecules of ATP per mole of glucose.

What various types of skeletal muscle fibres you know? On what basis are they classified?

Skeletal muscle fibres are classified into at least three types based on their metabolic needs and their mechanical performance.

Table 3.1 *Types of skeletal muscle fibres*

Property	Type I fibre	Type II fibre	Type III fibre
Mechanical performance	Slow	Fast	Fast
Metabolic need	Oxidative	Glycolytic	Oxidative
Colour	Red	White	Red

Most muscles are made up of both types of fibres. The myoglobin content gives the red colour to the Type I and Type III oxidative fibres.

How is skeletal muscle different from smooth and cardiac muscles?

Table 3.2 *Comparison between skeletal, cardiac and smooth muscle*

	Skeletal muscle	Cardiac muscle	Smooth muscle
Structure			
Motor endplate	Present	None	None
Mitochondria	Few	Many	Few
Sarcomere	Yes	Yes	None
Sarcoplasmic reticulum	Extensively developed	Well developed	Poorly developed
Syncytium	None	Yes	Yes
Function			
Pacemaker	No	Yes (fast)	Yes (slow)
Response	All or none	All or none	Graded
Tetanic contraction	Yes	No	Yes

Q3 Lung volumes

Can you draw a spirometry trace and tell me about the volumes and capacities.

The volumes are the residual volume, expiratory reserve volume, tidal volume and the inspiratory reserve volume.

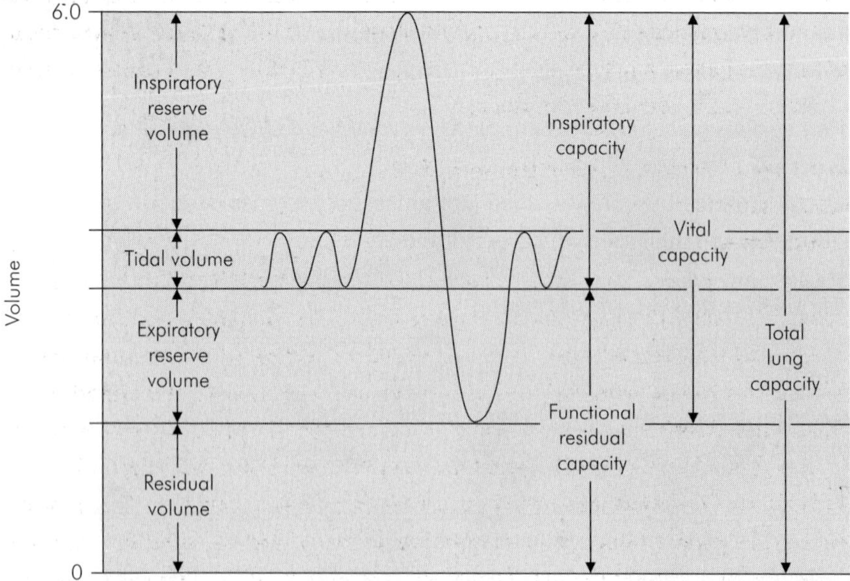

Figure 3.3 *Spirometry trace of lung volumes*

The capacities (which are the sum of volumes) include the functional residual capacity, vital capacity and the total lung capacity.

What is functional residual capacity (FRC) and what is its significance?
FRC is the volume of gas remaining in the lung at the end of a quiet expiration. It is the sum of residual volume and expiratory reserve volume. At the point of FRC the ability of the thoracic cage to expand and the elastic recoil of lung to collapse cancel each other and hence FRC represents a state of equilibrium.

Under normal conditions the gas in the FRC after a quite expiration acts as a reserve in the lung so that gas exchange continues to take place without interruption. The purpose of preoxygenation is to denitrogenate the FRC so that about 2500 ml of this capacity is filled with oxygen. This provides an additional resource for oxygen particularly if patient has to be apnoeic for a period. Thus any factor that decreases the FRC can increase the rate of desaturation.

Tell me the factors that affect the FRC.
- Age.
- Posture (reduced in supine position).
- Obesity.
- Pregnancy.
- Lung pathology (fibrosis, pulmonary oedema).
- Thoracic wall pathology (kyphosis, scoliosis, muscle weakness).

FRC is increased in chronic obstructive airway diseases and during positive intrathoracic pressure. FRC falls by about 25% in the supine position. Anaesthesia and surgical factors can further reduce the FRC mainly due to the compression of diaphragm by the abdominal contents.

What methods are available to measure FRC?
- Helium dilution.
- Body plethysmography.

In the first method helium is used because of its inert nature. It is neither soluble nor metabolised. The principle $V_1C_1 = V_2C_2$ is applied. The subject is made to breath through a spirometer with a known initial volume of fresh gas (V_1) with a known initial concentration of helium (C_1). This is continued until a state of equilibrium is reached where helium is diluted to a final concentration (C_2) in the larger combined volume V_2 (which is, V_1 + FRC). From the available values FRC can be derived.

In body plethysmography Boyle's gas law ($P_1V_1 = P_2V_2$) is applied. The subject makes an inspiratory effort in a closed chamber and the pressure and volume change before and after the inspiratory effort is measured. Applying the gas law FRC can be derived.

Pharmacology 3

Key topics: propofol/thiopental, antiepileptics, clinical trials

Q1 Intravenous induction agents

What intravenous induction agents are you familiar with?

Propofol, thiopental, etomidate, ketamine.

What are the properties of an ideal intravenous anaesthetic agent?

These can be categorised by physical, pharmacokinetic and pharmacodynamic properties.

- Physical
  - Soluble in water
  - Stable in solution-long shelf life
  - Stable when diluted
  - Stable in the presence of air, light and in room temperature
  - Should not encourage bacterial growth
- Pharmacokinetic
  - High oil/water solubility
  - Non-cumulative with infusion
  - Completely metabolised to inactive and non-toxic metabolites
  - Safe in the presence of liver/renal impairment
- Pharmacodynamic
  - No pain on injection
  - Induction in one-arm brain circulation time
  - Analgesic
  - Not epileptogenic, no increase in ICP
  - Muscle relaxation properties
  - No cardiovascular depression, cardiac irritation
  - No respiratory depression, bronchospasm
  - No histamine release
  - Safe in pregnancy and paediatrics

Tell me about propofol.

Propofol is a phenol type of intravenous induction agent. It is 2,6-di-isopropyl phenol. As it has minimal solubility in water it is formulated as an isotonic 1% or 2% emulsion in a mixture of 10% soyabean oil, 1.2% purified egg phosphatide, 2.25% glycerol, sodium hydroxide and water. This emulsion has a pH of 6–8.5 and a pKa of 11. At this pKa in the physiological pH (7.4) most of the drug is in un-ionised (active) form. It is used in a dose of 2–2.5 mg/kg for induction of anaesthesia.

What is the mechanism of action of propofol?

Propofol, like thiopental, acts on the GABA channels in the central nervous system (CNS). This effect is mediated via β-subunits of the $GABA_A$ receptors where the duration of opening of the chloride channels is increased.

Propofol may also have a role in regulating the (inhibitory) glycine receptor.

The other proposed mechanism of action is the reduction in the sodium channel opening times in the neuronal membranes in the CNS.

Can you tell about some unwanted effects of propofol?

- Pain on injection.
- Excitatory epileptiform movements; risk of convulsion when used in epileptics.
- Bradycardia and cardiovascular depression.
- Serious adverse reactions (1:50,000–100,000), possibly due to solubilising agents.
- Not licenced for use in pregnancy – high placental transfer and associated neonatal depression.
- Safety for prolonged infusion in paediatric population is questioned. It can lead to hyperlipidaemia, metabolic acidosis, myocardial failure and death.

What advantages of propofol have made it a popular intravenous anaesthetic agent?

- Rapid onset, clear headed-recovery.
- Fast 'street-fitness' in day care setting.
- Greater suppression of laryngeal reflexes making it more ideal for laryngeal mask airway insertion.
- Post-operative nausea and vomiting is extremely uncommon. Possible antiemetic effect.
- Elimination minimally affected by renal and hepatic function.
- Although context sensitive half time varies with duration of infusion, of the available intravenous anaesthetic agents it is minimally cumulative.

Can you compare and contrast propofol and thiopental?

Table 3.3 *Propofol and Thiopental*

	Propofol	Thiopental
Nature	A phenol. White, isotonic, neutral aqueous emulsion in soyabean oil, purified egg phosphatide, glycerol, NaOH and water	A barbiturate. Hygroscopic yellow powder with 6% $NaHCO_3$, reconstituted with water to 2.5% solution

(*Cont*)

Table 3.3 (*Continued*)

	Propofol	Thiopental
Properties		
Molecular weight	178	264
pH	6–8.5	10.8
pKa	11	7.6
Protein binding	98%	75%
Vd (l/kg)	3.3–5.5	1–4
Clearance (ml/min/kg)	20	1.4–5.7
Metabolism	Hepatic – Oxidation	Hepatic – conjugation
Elimination	Urine (<1% eliminated unchanged)	Urine (<1% eliminated unchanged)
Pharmacodynamics		
Onset	Rapid	Rapid
Recovery	Rapid	Relatively rapid; late recovery is delayed
t½ α 1 (initial rapid disposition to well perfused organs)	1–3 min	2–4 min
t½ α 2 (slower disposition to muscle and skin)	45 min	45–60 min
t½ β (elimination half-life)	1–5 h	5–10 h
Metabolites	2,6-diisopropylphenol glucuronide, 2,6-diisopropylquinol glucuronide	Thiopental carboxylic acid, hydroxythiopental, pentobarbital
CNS	ICP, CPP, $CMRO_2$, reduced, anticonvulsant, small risk of convulsions in epileptics	ICP, CPP, $CMRO_2$, reduced, anticonvulsant
CVS	Blood pressure and CO ↓, reduction in blood pressure is primarily due to ↓ systematic vascular (SV) and CO, Bradycardia can be profound	Blood pressure and CO ↓, reduction in blood pressure is primarily due to ↓ in systematic vascular resistance (SVR), compensatory tachycardia
Respiratory system	Respiratory depression, response to CO_2 ↓, greater suppression of laryngeal reflexes	Respiratory depression, response to CO_2 ↓, may cause laryngospasm/bronchoconstriction
Other effects	Pain on injection	Extravascular complications, risks associated with inadvertent intra-arterial injection

Q2 Clinical trials

What do you understand by a 'clinical trial'?

A clinical trial is the process whereby the efficacy and value of treatment or interventions are compared to a control group. The interventions may be treatments, diagnostic tests, screening programmes, etc.

What types of clinical trials are you aware of?

- Phased clinical trials.
- Cross over studies.
- Multi-centre trials.
- Meta-analysis.

Can you tell more about phased clinical trials? What are the various phases?

Phased clinical trials involve four phases. Before starting the clinical trial the compound to be tested needs to be synthesised in the laboratory and then undergo animal studies. Once the effects and obvious toxicity are identified with animal studies then the next step in the drug development is to enter into the clinical trial:

- *Phase I trial.* This is effected in a small group of either normal healthy volunteers or in patients who have failed to respond to existing conventional treatments. At this phase the main aim is to identify the maximum tolerated dose and to observe the pharmacokinetic properties of the given drug.
- *Phase II trial.* This is also carried out in a small group of patients with different dosage regimens. The motive is to again ascertain the potency, and identify obvious side effects. The results of this phase will form the basis to design the more organised in Phase III. Neither Phase I nor Phase II is randomised.
- *Phase III trial.* Based on Phase II an optimal dose and frequency is determined and a proper randomised control trial is done. There is a placebo group (receiving no intervention), control group (receiving an existing conventional intervention) and the study group (receiving the newer intervention of interest). If the therapeutic efficacy is acceptable, a drug licence is granted at this stage.
- *Phase IV trial.* Also called post-marketing surveillance, this phase runs for a longer period in order to identify the long-term safety and efficacy of the newer intervention.

What do you mean by meta-analysis?

Meta-analysis is pooling the data from a number of smaller individual trials and analysing the effect of the given intervention. The aim is to enhance the statistical precision which smaller studies may not provide. The results are usually expressed as 'confidence intervals'.

The limitation of meta-analysis is that combining various studies with potential bias may draw erroneous results.

How can you minimise bias?

- *Randomisation*: Ensuring that every participant in the study has the same chance of ending up in any of the treatment groups.
- *Blinding*: A clinical trial should ideally have a 'double-blind design' where both patient and investigator are unaware of the intervention identity.

Can you outline the various steps involved in planning a clinical trial?

1. *Aim of the study*: What is the question, what is the best way to get the answer? Will the results make a difference and create a change?
2. *Review of literature*: Has similar work been done before (to avoid 're-discovering' things).
3. *Study design*: Inclusion, exclusion criteria, methods, consent, early involvement of statistician to calculate the 'power', the number needed to identify a statistically and clinically important difference, duration of study, funding.
4. *Ethical committee approval*: Patient information leaflet, consent form; ethical committee approval is mandatory before starting the trial.
5. *Patients and methods*: Protocols, randomisation, blinding.
6. *Data collection.*
7. *Data analysis*: Statistical tests.
8. *Presentation of results.*
9. *Publication.*

Q3 Anticonvulsants

Can you classify anticonvulsant drugs?

Types of anticonvulsants are:

- Hydantoins (phenytoin)
- Barbiturates (phenobarbital)
- Succinimides (ethosuximide)
- Benzodiazepines (diazepam, lorazepam)
- Miscellaneous agents (carbemazepine, primidone, magnesium sulphate, lamotrigine, gabapentin).

What is the mechanism of action of anticonvulsant drugs?

Exact mode and site of action of these drugs are still unknown at the molecular level.

Main pharmacological effects are as follows:

- To increase motor cortex threshold to reduce its response to incoming electrical or chemical stimulation.
- To depress or reduce the spread of a seizure discharge from its focus (origin) by depressing synaptic transport or decreasing nerve conduction.

The proposed mechanisms are:

1. *GABA facilitation*: benzodiazepines, barbiturates
2. *GABA agonism*: progabide
3. *GABA transaminase inactivation*: valproate, vigabatrin
4. *Fast sodium channel blockade*: phenytoin
5. *Presynaptic sodium channel stabilisation*: lamotrigine, valproate.

Tell me more about phenytoin.

Phenytoin is a membrane stabiliser, an antiepileptic drug with local anaesthetic and antiarrhythmic properties. It acts on the fast sodium channels thereby interfering with depolarisation during the action potential. It may also interfere with calcium entry. Cells that are firing respectively at high frequency are blocked preferentially which permits discrimination between epileptic and physiological activity.

Phenytoin can be given by mouth or in the form of intravenous injection but should not be given intramuscularly. It is used in status epilepticus and in tonic–clonic seizures. It has a very narrow therapeutic index and hence the level has to be regularly monitored. Although it has been used in chronic pain conditions with a neuropathic element, because of its unwanted effects profile its role is now limited. Adverse effects include gum hyperplasia, coarsening of facial features, hirsuitism, Dupuytren's contracture, pseudolymphoma, megaloblastic anaemia and fetal malformations.

Once administered it follows zero-order kinetics, therefore half-life is dose dependent. About 85% is bound to protein. Phenytoin is a potent enzyme inducer and has several drug interactions.

What is gabapentin and how does it act?

Gabapentin is an amino acid. Originally introduced as an antiepileptic, it is now extensively used in the management of neuropathic pain in chronic pain patients. The relative safety over a wide dosage range and minimal drug interactions have made it an attractive agent in chronic pain management. It is used as an adjunct in treatment of partial seizures.

The exact mechanism of action is not clearly known but there are various postulations:

- Modulates voltage sensitive calcium channels.
- Inhibition of voltage sensitive sodium channels.
- Increased synthesis of brain GABA (inhibitory neurotransmitter).
- Inhibition synthesis of glutamate (excitatory neurotransmitter).
- Increased 5-HT secretion.
- Competition with certain amino acids (leucine, isoleucine, valine, phenylalanine) for specific amino acid transmembrane transporter.

Clinical 3

Key topics: renal failure, atrial fibrillation, blood transfusion

Q1 A 64-year-old female with chronic renal failure (CRF) presents for multiple wisdom teeth extraction.

What are the problems associated with CRF that are of anaesthetic concern?

CRF is associated with significantly reduced renal function and has effects on several systems in the body. Problems include:

- *Cardiovascular system*: hypertension, prone to ischaemic heart disease, pericardial effusion in advanced cases, altered sympathetic response due to antihypertensive drugs.
- *Respiratory system*: pulmonary oedema, pleural effusion, prone to respiratory infections.
- *Gastrointestinal tract*: uraemic gastropathy, loss of appetite, cachexia, risk of regurgitation.
- *CNS*: encephalopathy, uraemic confusional state.
- *Metabolic*: acidosis, unpredictable intravascular fluid volume, hyperkalaemia, hypermagnesaemia, hypocalcaemia, hyponatraemia.
- *Blood*: anaemia, platelet dysfunction.
- *Pharmacology*: altered pharmacokinetics and pharmacodynamics.

The conditions that lead to CRF (e.g. diabetes mellitus, hypertension) may influence the choice and conduct of anaesthesia.

What are the causes of anaemia in renal failure?

- Nutritional (poor appetite).
- Decreased renin synthesis.
- Bone marrow suppression.
- Decreased red cell life span.
- Bleeding tendency.

These are the blood results of this patient:

Hb 7 g/dl	Platelets 272 × 10^9/l	Urea 15.6 mmol/l
Creatinine 213 μmol/l	Na^+ 132 mmol/l	K^+ 5.9 mmol/l

Can you comment on these results?

She is anaemic. Her urea and creatinine are elevated and her electrolyte abnormalities include hyperkalaemia and hyponatraemia.

Why are you concerned about hyperkalaemia?

Potassium is the most important ion in maintenance of transcellular membrane potential. Hyperkalaemia can lead to life threatening arrhythmias including ventricular fibrillation. The ECG changes include tall T-waves and wide QRS complexes.

Can you tell me some other causes of hyperkalaemia?

- *Spurious*: due to haemolysed blood sample, also can be seen in thrombocytosis, massive leucocytosis and vigorous exercise.
- *Decreased excretion*: renal failure, aldosterone deficiency, Addison's disease.
- *Drugs*: such as potassium-sparing diuretics (amiloride, spiranolctone), ACE inhibitors and non-steroidal anti-inflammation drugs.
- *Release of K^+ from the cells*: acidosis, drugs such as succinylcholine (suxamethonium), beta blockers, malignant hyperthermia, massive blood transfusion and incompatible blood transfusion.

What are the various measures available to treat hyperkalaemia?

1 Measures to protect the heart: calcium chloride.
2 Measures to redistribute the serum K^+ are:
   - Beta 2 agonists.
   - Dextrose and insulin to drive potassium inside the cells.
   - $NaHCO_3$.
   - Hyperventilation in ventilated patients. Alkalinisation of the blood causes H^+ to come out of the cells to neutralise the pH. To maintain the electrical neutrality K^+ enters inside the cells.

3 Measures to eliminate K^+ from body are:
- Resins: sodium and calcium resins.
- Haemodialysis or haemofiltration.

Her platelet count is 272 × 10^9/l. Are you happy that her bleeding time will be normal?

No. Although the numbers are normal, there may yet be platelet dysfunction that can lead to an abnormal bleeding tendency.

She is anaemic. Do you think preoperative blood transfusion will be safe for her?

In general, CRF patients have long-standing anaemia and they tolerate it well. Also dental extraction is not often associated with abnormal blood loss to warrant blood transfusion. So as long as the patient is not symptomatic, transfusion is unnecessary and may be harmful in terms of circulatory overload. In symptomatic patients erythropoietin can be of some use.

If this patient is on haemodialysis what additional details would you like to get?

- Where is the fistula?
- When she was last filtered?
- What were her urea and electrolytes after filtration?

If very recently filtered she would have been heparinised. Therefore, look for activated partial thromboplastin time (APTT).

Recent haemofiltration can render her relatively hypovolaemic. Therefore, careful assessment of her fluid status is important.

What is the half-life of heparin? How long should you wait following heparinisation?

The half-life of heparin is about 45–90 min. The clinical effects of heparin on clotting last for up to 4 h.

Outline the salient points in intraoperative anaesthetic management of this patient.

- Avoid intravenous access and non-invasive blood pressure (NIBP) in the arm having the atrioventricular (AV) fistula.
- Consider the aspiration risk.
- Care in case of nasotracheal intubation due of risk of bleeding.
- Choose drugs that have a predictable effect in renal failure and do not depend on renal elimination.

- Meticulous fluid management. Normal daily allowance should be noted preoperatively. Intraoperative fluid administration should include the maintenance fluid and replacement of blood loss. Avoid potassium-containing fluids.
- Prepare for abnormal bleeding from extraction site.

What are your thoughts about using suxamethonium in renal failure patients?
The concern is the transient rise in serum potassium level following suxamethonium that is dangerous in pre-existing hyperkalaemia. If the preoperative levels are normal and if the clinical situation warrants, suxamethonium can be safely used.

What about using opioids in renal failure?
Remifentanil is ultra-short acting and its metabolism is independent of renal function. Short acting opioids like alfentanil and fentanyl are safe in single doses, but multiple doses and increased dosage can lead to delayed respiratory depression. Longer acting drugs like pethidine and morphine have active metabolites that are excreted through kidneys. Norpethidine a metabolite of pethidine, is epileptogenic. The metabolite of morphine, morphine-6-glucuronide, has an analgesic and sedative effect that can make morphine unpredictably long acting in these patients.

Q2 Critical incident: arrhythmia

You have induced general anaesthesia and secured the airway with a nasotracheal tube. Anaesthesia is being maintained with sevoflurane, oxygen and nitrous oxide. At the beginning of the surgery the surgeon has infiltrated using lidocaine with epinephrine.

Half way through the procedure you notice the heart rate is going up. What will you do now?
Check the heart rate and rhythm, also quickly check the blood pressure and SaO_2.

This is the rhythm and rate is about 120/min. How will you react?

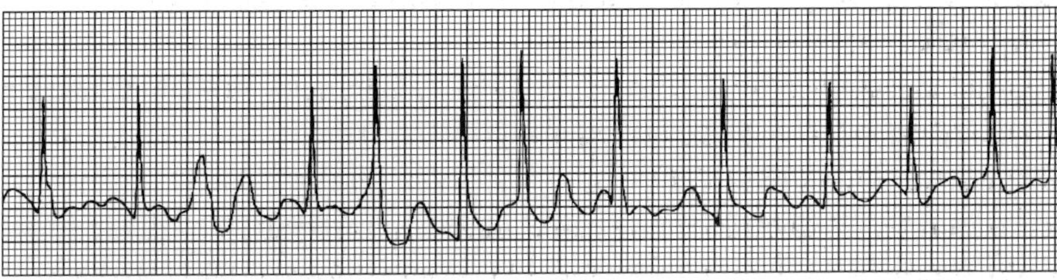

Figure 3.4 *ECG rhythm strip, AF*

The rhythm shows atrial fibrillation (AF):

- Inform the surgeon and stop the surgery.
- Call for help and in the mean time attempt to treat the patient.
- Check for pulse, blood pressure, SaO_2.
- Increase inspired oxygen.
- Amiodarone 300 mg in 5% dextrose intravenously over 1 h followed by 900 mg over 24 h.
- Alternatively a beta blocker (metoprolol 1–2 mg/min, maximum 5 mg) or digoxin 250–500 μg as a slow intravenous infusion if blood pressure is stable.
- If sinus rhythm is not restored with above measures or if there is haemodynamic instability then cardioversion should be considered.

As you draw up amiodarone you notice that the heart rate has gone up to 170/min and blood pressure is 68/40 mmHg.

Give synchronised direct current shock (cardioversion)
100 J, 200 J, 360 J (monophasic defibrillator)

What conditions can predispose to AF?

AF can be due to (mnemonic: RHEUMATIC):

R: Rheumatic heart disease
H: Hypoxia, hypotension
E: Electrolyte disturbances (hypokalaemia, hypomagnesaemia)
U: Wolff–Parkinson–White syndrome
M: Myocarditis
A: Airway diseases (COAD, pneumonia)
T: Thyrotoxicosis
I: Ischaemic heart disease
C: Cardiomyopathy

What are the likely causes for AF in this patient?

- Associated ischaemic heart disease.
- Use of epinephrine along with lidocaine.
- Electrolyte imbalance.

How much epinephrine will you allow the surgeon to use?

Surgeons usually use 2% lidocaine with 1:80,000 epinephrine.

1 ml of this mixture contains 12.5 μg of epinephrine; maximum 100 μg of epinephrine can be infiltrated over period of 10 min. In this patient as there is increased risk of arrhythmias the dose should be reduced.

Q3 Blood transfusion

What you understand by autologous blood transfusion?

Autologous transfusion means transfusing the patient's own blood to correct the blood loss during surgery.

One of the following three methods can be used for autologous transfusion:

1. *Predonation*: Blood is collected from the patient 4–5 weeks prior to the surgery. The patient's haemoglobin can be improved with supplemental iron.
2. *Acute normovolaemic haemodilution*: Immediately before the surgery one or more units of blood is withdrawn from the patient and the intravascular volume is replaced by colloids or crystalloids.
3. *Intraoperative blood salvage*: Blood is collected from the operating field, washed and then transfused back to the patient.

How would you manage massive haemorrhage?

The management strategy would be: Airway, Breathing, Circulation, summon help.

The important principles are:

- To replenish the circulating volume immediately (with crystalloids, colloids)
- To improve the oxygen carrying capacity (with blood)
- To achieve surgical control of bleeding
- To improve the quality of blood (fresh frozen plasma, platelets)
- Once stabilised patient will require more intensive monitoring in a controlled environment.

What is massive blood transfusion?

Massive blood transfusion has variably been defined as follows:

- When blood is transfused at a rate more than 10% of the volume in less than 10 min.
- If greater than 50% of the patient's blood volume requires replacement in a short time.
- Replacement of the patient's total blood volume with stored blood in less than 24 h.

What are the complications of blood transfusion?

Complications of blood transfusion can broadly be classified into immunological and non-immunological, immediate and delayed.

- *Immediate immunological*:
  - Haemolytic transfusion reactions (often due to ABO incompatibility)
  - Febrile non-haemolytic transfusion reactions (due to recipient antileucocyte antibodies)

- Anaphylaxis (related to IgA deficiency in the recipient)
- Urticaria (due to plasma proteins)

- *Immediate non-immunological*:
  - Metabolic effects: Acid–base changes, hyperkalaemia, reduced ionised calcium
  - Citrate toxicity
  - Hypothermia
  - Dilutional coagulopathy
  - Congestive cardiac failure
- *Delayed immunological*:
  - Delayed haemolytic transfusion reactions
  - Delayed febrile reactions
  - Transfusion related acute lung injury (TRALI)
  - Transfusion associated graft versus host disease (TA-GVHD)
- *Delayed non-immunological*:
  - Viral infection: HIV, hepatitis C, hepatitis B, hepatitis A.
  - Bacterial infection: Contamination of red cells with *Yersinia enterocolitica*; contamination of platelets with *Staphylococcus epidermidis, Klebsiella pneumoniae.*
  - Parasite infection: Malaria.

Physics, clinical measurement and safety 3

Key topics: temperature measurement, vaporiser, biological signals, monitoring depth of anaesthesia

Q1 Temperature measurement

How may temperature be measured?

Methods may be electrical and non-electrical.

- *Non-electrical*:
  - Mercury thermometer
  - Alcohol thermometer
  - Dial thermometer
- *Electrical*:
  - Resistance thermometer
  - Thermistor
  - Thermocouple

What are the limitations of a mercury thermometer for use in the operating theatre?

- Long response time of 2–3 min for equilibration.
- Limited sites for measurement. Rectal measurements may be inaccurate owing to slowness and presence of faecal material.
- Risk of rectal perforation in neonates.
- Rigid with risk of breakage and trauma. Toxic.

What is the principle behind the resistance thermometer?

The resistance of metal increases linearly with temperature. Simple devices can either be a resistance thermometer containing a platinum wire, battery and an ammeter calibrated to indicate temperature or incorporated into Wheatstone bridge circuit containing an array of resistors to improve accuracy.

How does a thermistor work? What are its advantages and disadvantages?

A thermistor has a little bead of semiconductor (metal oxide) whose resistance falls exponentially as temperature increases.

- *Advantages*:
  - Convenient to use in theatres because of its compactness and fast response.
  - Although the change is non-linear it can be manufactured so that over the working range it is almost linear.
  - Thermistor undergoes greater change in resistance over the clinical range of temperature than the resistance thermometer.
- *Disadvantage*:
  - Calibration is liable to change over time ('drift') or if subjected to extremes of temperature as in sterilisation.

What is the principle behind the thermocouple?

In a junction of two dissimilar metals a voltage develops, the magnitude of which depends upon the temperature at the junction. This is called Seebeck effect.

There is a reference junction kept at constant temperature and a measuring junction that acts as a probe.

What are the advantages of the electrical methods over the non-electrical ones?

Electrical probes have shorter response time of 1–15 s (smaller probes have a smaller heat capacity than large probes).

Greater selection of sites for measurement.

What are the sites available for temperature measurement?

- *Nasopharynx*: approximates to brain temperature.
- *Ear*: risk of drum perforation.

- *Lower oesophagus*: approximates to cardiac temperature (but recording tip should be not too high to be cooled by inspired gases in lower trachea).
- *Pulmonary artery*: measures core temperature.
- *Rectum*
- *Urinary bladder*
- *Skin*: peripheral-core temperature gradient may give a useful index of adequacy of peripheral perfusion.

Q2 Vaporisers

What factors determine the degree of vaporisation of a liquid in a vaporiser?

- Gas flow through the vaporising chamber (splitting ratio).
- Surface area available for vaporisation.
- Temperature.
- Volatility of the liquid concerned.

What are the characters of an ideal vaporiser?

- Should have an accurate performance over a wide range of gas flow (flow compensated).
- Performance should not be affected by ambient temperature or the temperature of liquid (temperature compensated).
- Should have low resistance and should be suitable to use both inside and outside the circle system.
- Should be economic to use and durable with minimum servicing requirement.

Why does the temperature fall during vaporisation?

For the change of liquid to vapour state, heat is required – latent heat of vaporisation. This heat is taken up from the liquid itself or from the container. Hence the liquid temperature falls.

Define latent heat of vaporisation?

Latent heat of vaporisation, is the heat required to convert 1 kg of substance from the liquid phase to the gaseous phase at a given temperature expressed in J/kg.

What do you mean by specific heat capacity?

Specific heat capacity of a substance is the heat required to raise the temperature of 1 kg of that substance by 1 kelvin (K), expressed in $J/kg\ K^{-1}$ (where the temperature in K = °C + 273.15).

What physical principles are involved in constructing a plenum vaporiser?

- Fresh gas flow is split into two using splitting ratio and a desired volume of gas is passed through the vaporising chamber using a positive pressure.
- Surface area of the liquid which is in contact with carrier gas is maximised so that all the gas passing through the vaporising chamber is saturated with the vapour.
- A temperature compensating mechanism to adjust the splitting ratio so that a constant concentration of the vapour is maintained is needed.

Can you name some methods that have been used to increase the vaporisation?

- Use of wicks to increase the surface area of contact.
- Directing the gas flow on to the surface of liquid or bubbling through the liquid using a plunger as in Boyle's bottle.
- Baffles to repeatedly redirect the gas flow on to the surface of the liquid.
- Maintaining temperature of the liquid or compensating for fall in temperature so that the degree of vaporisation does not fall with fall in temperature.

What mechanisms have been used in vaporisers to compensate for the changes in temperature? How do they work?

The mechanisms include temperature-sensitive valves of different types. Examples: bimetallic strips, ether-filled bellows or metal rods.

A bimetallic strip is made up of two dissimilar metals with different coefficient of thermal expansion; with decreasing temperature, it bends and allows more carrier gas to pass through the vaporising chamber.

Ether-filled bellows and metal rods contract with decreasing temperature. The principle remains the same in that the splitting ratio is altered and the vapour concentration maintained.

Vaporisers are made of materials with high specific heat capacity to minimise heat loss.

What is the effect of using a ventilator that produces back pressure in the system?

Back pressure develops during the inspiratory phase which forces gas from the outlet port back into the vaporising chamber (pumping). This can lead to an undue increase in delivered vapour concentration.

How can this be avoided?

- By using downstream flow restrictors to prevent back flow.
- By constructing bypass channel and vaporising chamber of equal size, so that even if there is a back flow due to pressure, the gas equally divides between the two chambers and the vapour concentration is unaffected.

- By increasing the length of inlet tube. This will avoid retrograde mixing of the vapour rich gases in the vaporising chamber with the fresh gases in the bypass chamber.

What safety features are incorporated into modern vaporisers?

- Accurate at low flows and over wide range of gas flow: 0.5–15 l/min.
- Antispill mechanism; can be tilted to 180° or tipped upside down.
- Interlocking system; so that even when more than one vaporiser is mounted on the back bar of anaesthetic machine, only one can be used at a time.
- Compensation for back pressure and pressure fluctuations.
- Keyed filler: colour coded: purple: isoflurane; yellow: sevoflurane; blue: desflurane.
- Safety lock facility (locked on the back bar).

How does a desflurane vaporiser differ from the rest?

Tec 6 vaporisers are specifically designed for desflurane which boils at 23.5°C and has a high saturated vapour pressure (SVP) of 88 kPa. Desflurane is heated to 39°C in the vaporising chamber, and the SVP increases to about 200 kPa. SVP varies with temperature. Therefore, by heating desflurane to a constant temperature and increasing the SVP a constant vapour concentration from the vaporising chamber is ensured. A pressure-reducing valve reduces the pressure equal to that of carrier gas. There is a differential pressure transducer which senses the pressure of carrier gas and adjusts the pressure-reducing valve accordingly. A control valve (concentration dial) regulates the flow of desflurane gas into the fresh gas flow.

Q3 Biological potentials

What is the EMG?

EMG stands for electromyogram. It is the recording of muscle potentials from surface electrodes or needle electrodes. A graph is obtained with voltage on the y-axis and time on the x-axis.

What is the difference between ECG potentials and EMG potentials?

Duration of the action potential is shorter in skeletal muscle, about 5–10 ms. Whereas in ECG it is more than 200 ms. The waveform of EMG is a sharp spike unlike the complex pattern in ECG. The size of ECG signals is about 1–2 mV. In EMG this can vary from about 100 μV to many mV. The frequency range of ECG is 0–100 Hz. It is 0–1000 Hz for EMG.

Can you explain the process of obtaining and recording biological signals?

It is explained using a 'black box concept'. The process has three components: detection, amplification and recording or display.

Electrodes are used in the detection of potentials. Biological signals cause a small current to flow through an electrode. This creates some chemical changes in the electrode and generates a potential.

The amplifier used is usually '*differential amplifier*' that measures the potential difference from two sources. This 'differential amplification' can eliminate the interference common to both the electrodes. This ability is described as '*common mode rejection*'. The ratio of the voltage at the output of the amplifier to the signal voltage at the input is known as the '*gain*' of the amplifier. The range of frequencies over which the amplification is relatively constant is known as the '*bandwidth*' of the amplifier.

The recording or the display can be with galvanometer recorders, potentiometric recorders or with cathode ray tubes. With modern technology, integrated circuits are incorporated in the system and biological potentials can be displayed as a set of figures.

How is an ECG trace displayed on the monitor screen?

Usually follows the principle of a cathode ray tube. Hot cathode produces an electron beam which passes through two deflecting devices, one of which deflects the beam horizontally on the x-axis and the other plate deflects the beam vertically on the y-axis. The beams then strike the fluorescent screen to produce a trace on a fluorescent screen which glows when struck by an electron beam. Biological action potentials such as ECG deflect the beam in the y-direction producing a vertical deflection over time. The system is calibrated so that 1 mV signal gives 1 cm vertical displacement of the trace.

What is ECT? What does an ECT stimulator do?

ECT stands for electroconvulsive therapy. A current of 850 mA is passed through the brain in the form of brief pulses of 1.25 ms at 26 Hz. The total duration of stimulus is 2–5 s. Two electrodes, one for each temple, are used and this induces cerebral seizure that has therapeutic benefit.

How do you monitor depth of anaesthesia?

Depth of anaesthesia can be monitored by:

1 Clinical parameters: autonomic responses, Guedel staging.
2 Using specialised equipment:
   - Isolated forearm technique.
   - Frontalis muscle activity.
   - Lower oesophageal contractility.
   - Monitoring electroencephalogram EEG with various modifications-evoked potentials, compressed spectral array, bispectral index (BIS).

What is the EEG?

EEG is the abbreviation for electroencephalogram. It involves surface recording of electrical potentials arising from the cerebral cortex.

Why are we not using EEG routinely?

A vast quantity of information is obtained from EEG and is difficult to interpret. The generated pattern also depends on the anaesthetic agents – different agents produce different patterns. EEG is also affected by various pathophysiological events such as hypoxia, hypotension and hypercarbia.

What are the various frequency bands in the EEG signal and what happens to EEG with increasing depth of anaesthesia?

The four commonly recognised bands in EEG include α (8–13 Hz), β (>13 Hz) δ (<4 Hz), and θ (4–7 Hz). With increasing depth of anaesthesia there is decrease in the frequency and amplitude of the EEG signals.

What is compressed spectral array?

Raw EEG is difficult to analyse. Compressed spectral array gives a three dimensional picture with amplitude on the y-axis, frequency on the x-axis and time on the z-axis. To do this several segments of EEG activity are recorded and the 'power' contained within different frequencies (α, β, δ and θ) is calculated. This is displayed as series of troughs and peaks. As the depth of anaesthesia increases the 'power' shifts to the lower frequencies and hence becomes a guide to assess the degree of cerebral suppression.

What do you mean by the terms spectral edge frequency and median frequency?

As interpreting EEG needs special skill and training its routine use is limited. To overcome this problem the analogue signal can be converted to a digital value which is easy to use in the assessment of depth of anaesthesia. Two of this numerical values used clinically are the spectral edge frequency and the median frequency.

Spectral edge is that frequency below which 95% of the power in compressed spectral array is contained. With increasing anaesthetic depth, spectral edge frequency decreases.

Median frequency is the mid-point of the power distribution in compressed spectral array. This is claimed to be a more reliable indicator of the depth of anaesthesia than the spectral edge.

What is BIS?

An algorithm was developed by studying various components of EEG in healthy volunteers and correlating the EEG pattern with clinical measures of anaesthetic depth. The monitor generates a number called BIS on a continuous scale of 0–100; 100 represents normal cortical activity and 0 represents no cortical activity.

BIS values of 40–60 imply adequate depth.

BIS represents an integrated measure of cerebral activity. It incorporates several processed EEG parameters such as bispectral analysis and power spectral analysis. The continuous EEG recording is sectioned into segments called '*epochs*'. The epochs undergo Fourier analysis.

What do you mean by Fourier analysis?

Fourier analysis is breakdown of complex waveforms into simple sine wave constituents.

SOE 4

Physiology 4

Key topics: shunt, hypoxic pulmonary vasoconstriction, baroreceptors, Valsalva manoeuvre, nerve action potential

Q1 Respiratory physiology

Can you write down the alveolar gas equation?

$$P_AO_2 = F_IO_2(P_B - P_{SVP}) - P_ACO_2/RQ$$

where P_AO_2 is the oxygen tension in the alveoli, P_B is the barometric pressure, P_{SVP} is the saturated water vapour pressure and RQ is the respiratory quotient which is normally 0.8.

What do you understand by the 'oxygen cascade'?
The oxygen cascade describes the stepwise fall in the oxygen tension starting from inspired air until it reaches the tissues. A concentration gradient is thus established and oxygen transport is maintained down this gradient.

What is the normal alveolar-arterial oxygen tension gradient? Why does this gradient exist?
In normal conditions there is a difference of 0.5–1 kPa in oxygen tension ($P_AO_2 - P_aO_2$) across the alveolar membrane. This is because of ventilation perfusion mismatch and is also due to venous admixture – shunt.

What do you mean by shunt? What contributes to normal physiological shunting?
Shunt refers to the part of the blood which does not take part in gas exchange. Bronchial veins directly drain to pulmonary veins and thebesian veins directly drain to the left ventricle and these contribute to the physiological shunt.

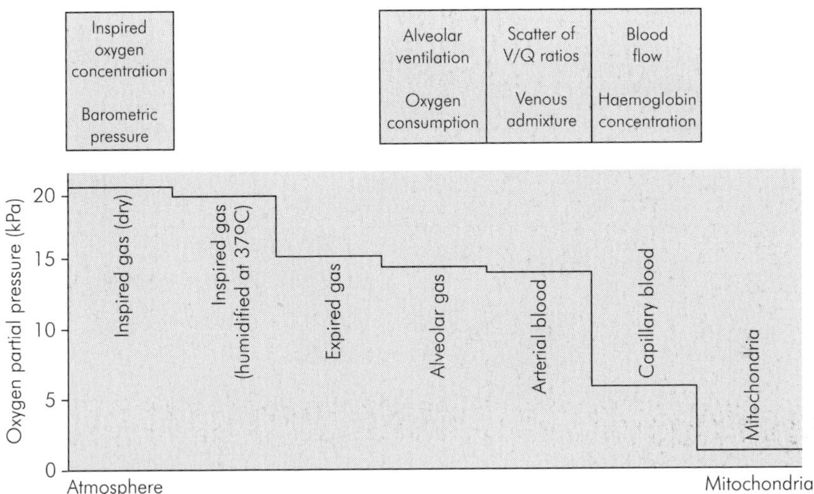

Figure 4.1 *Oxygen cascade*

Can you name some pathological causes of increased shunt?

Primary cardiac pathology: Intracardiac shunts, pulmonary atrioventricular (AV) fistula.

Primary pulmonary pathology: Pneumonia, acute respiratory distress syndrome (ARDS), bronchial obstruction, one-lung ventilation.

Depending on age the normal shunt fraction can vary between 2% and 5%. Shunt from 5% to 10% may not carry clinical significance. If the shunt fraction exceeds 30%, even increasing inspired oxygen to 100% will not improve arterial hypoxemia.

Derive the shunt equation. Can you explain it with a simple diagram?

- The total oxygen content of blood leaving the lungs is equal to the product of cardiac output (Q_T) and arterial oxygen content (C_aO_2).
- It is apparent from the diagram that this total oxygen content is contributed by two components namely $Q_S \times C_VO_2$ and $(Q_T - Q_S) \times C_CO_2$.

Therefore,

$$Q_T \times C_aO_2 = Q_S \cdot C_VO_2 + (Q_T - Q_S) \cdot C_CO_2$$

$$Q_T \times C_aO_2 = Q_S \cdot C_VO_2 + Q_T \cdot C_CO_2 - Q_S \cdot C_CO_2$$

Rearranging the equation,

$$Q_S \cdot C_CO_2 - Q_S \cdot C_VO_2 = Q_T \cdot C_CO_2 - Q_T \cdot C_aO_2$$

$$Q_S \cdot (C_CO_2 - C_VO_2) = Q_T \cdot (C_CO_2 - C_aO_2)$$

Hence shunt $Q_S/Q_T = C_CO_2 - C_aO_2/C_CO_2 - C_VO_2$.

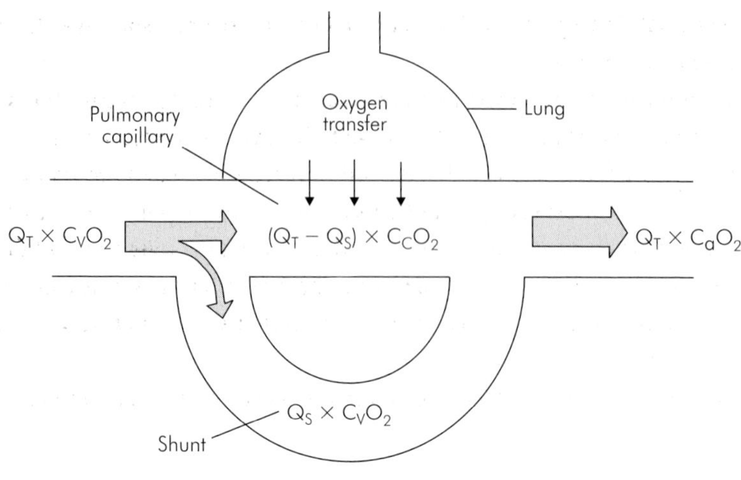

C_aO_2 = arterial oxygen content
C_VO_2 = mixed venous content
C_CO_2 = pulmonary capillary oxygen content
Q_T = cardiac output
Q_S = shunt flow
$(Q_T - Q_S)$ = pulmonary capillary blood flow

Figure 4.2 *Diagram of shunt in the lung*

What do you mean by hypoxic pulmonary vasoconstriction?

Hypoxic pulmonary vasoconstriction (HPV) is a protective physiological mechanism to maintain an optimal ventilation perfusion match by diverting the pulmonary blood flow from poorly ventilated areas to better ventilated areas. There is a reflex vasoconstriction of small pulmonary arterioles of 30–50 μm calibre in response to low alveolar oxygen tension of less than 11–13 kPa. This plays an important role in the fetus where it increases the pulmonary vascular resistance and reduces the pulmonary blood flow.

What factors modify HPV?

It is potentiated by acidosis and by drugs such as cyclo-oxygenase inhibitors, propranolol and almitrine.

It is attenuated by hypocapnia, volatile anaesthetic agents, vasodilators and bronchodilators.

What is the mechanism for HPV?

The exact mechanism is not known. It has been demonstrated in isolated lungs so does not depend upon the vessel wall innervation.

Q2 Valsalva manoeuvre

What are baroreceptors? Where are they located and what are their functions?

These are stretch receptors located in the walls of blood vessels and heart chambers. They are stimulated by the distension and play a crucial role in short term control of arterial blood pressure. They can be high- or low-pressure stretch receptors depending on their location.

The high-pressure stretch receptors are located in the carotid sinus and aortic arch. These receptors are progressively stimulated above a mean arterial pressure of 60 mmHg with a maximum effect at 180 mmHg. Afferent impulses are transmitted through branches of glossopharyngeal nerve (carotid sinus nerve) and vagus nerve (from aortic arch) to the medulla (which has vasomotor centre and cardio-inhibitory centre). A rise in blood pressure increases the firing rate and causes reflex inhibition of vasomotor centre and excitation of cardio-inhibitory centre resulting in lowering of blood pressure.

There are other stretch receptors located in the atria, ventricles and pulmonary vessels.

What is a Valsalva manoeuvre? Can you describe the physiological changes during the Valsalva manoeuvre?

The Valsalva manoeuvre is classically described a forced expiration against a closed glottis (though, in practice, it is creation of a positive intrathoracic pressure). It involves production of a square wave rise in intrathoracic pressure of 40 mmHg for duration of 10 s. The changes can be analysed in four stages. See Table 4.1.

What happens in autonomic neuropathy?

In autonomic neuropathy, there is a persistent fall in the blood pressure following a positive intrathoracic pressure. There is no reflex tachycardia. On release of the intrathoracic pressure the overshooting of the blood pressure does not happen. This implies an impaired baroreceptor reflex.

Q3 Nerve action potential

What happens when you stimulate a nerve cell?

Nerve cells have a low threshold for excitation. When stimulated two types of responses are produced.

- Local non-propagated potential known as a synaptic potential.
- Propagated potential known as an action potential.

Can you draw a nerve action potential and describe the potential changes during an action potential in a nerve cell?

At resting state, inside of the cell is negative in relation to the outside of the cell. This is known as *resting membrane potential*, which is –70 mV. When the nerve is stimulated, Na^+ ions move into the cell, which initiates depolarisation. After an initial 15 mV depolarisation, the rate of depolarisation increases. The point at

Table 4.1 *Valsalva manoeuvre*

Phase	Intrathoracic pressure	Blood pressure	Heart rate	Comments
I	Sharp increase in intrathoracic pressure	Transient increase in blood pressure due to (a) transmission of intrathoracic pressure in the aorta and (b) compression of pulmonary veins, forcing their contents into left atrium thereby increasing cardiac output	No change	Direct effect of transmitted pressure
II	Sustained holding of the positive intrathoracic pressure	Decrease in blood pressure due to reduction of venous return. Reflex vasoconstriction and tachycardia restore blood pressure towards normal	Increases	Baroreceptor reflex is coming into play
III	Sudden drop in the intrathoracic pressure	Drop in the blood pressure	No change	Fall in aortic pressure, venous return fills the pulmonary vessels and central veins rather than contributing to cardiac output
IV	Normal intrathoracic pressure	Overshoot in blood pressure as vasoconstriction still persists but venous return and cardiac output have returned to normal	Bradycardia (increased blood pressure causes reflex bradycardia and vasodilatation to restore blood pressure to normal)	-

which this change occurs is known as *threshold potential*. Then the potential rapidly overshoots above the isopotential line to approximately +35 mV. At this stage sodium diffusion is terminated and potassium diffuses out of the cell. This reverses the process and is known as repolarisation. When repolarisation is about 70%

complete, the process slows down and the resting potential is reached. The rapid rise and fall in potential difference is known as the spike potential.

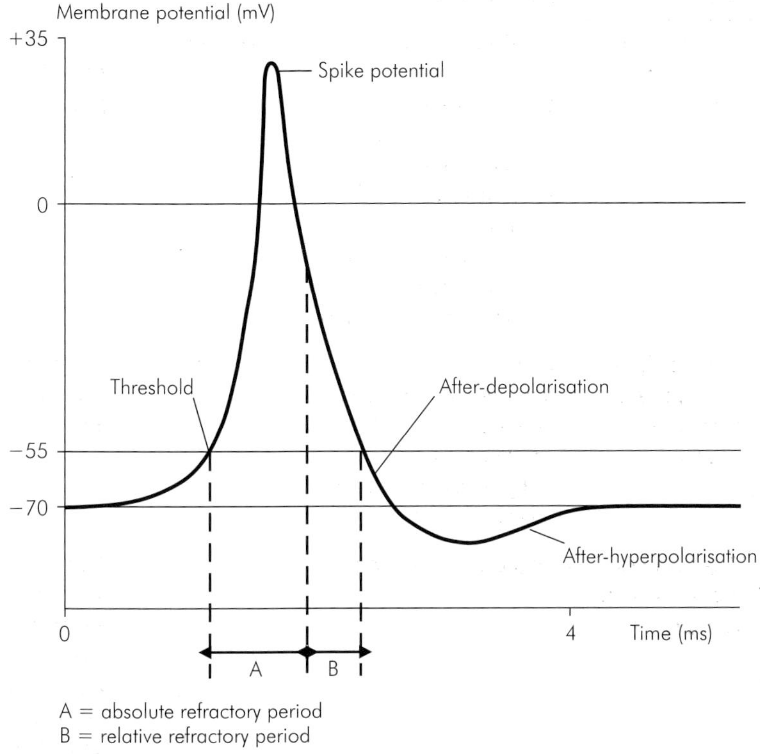

Figure 4.3 *Different phases of an action potential*

Show me on the diagram the absolute refractory period and relative refractory period.

Absolute refractory period is the period from the time of threshold level until repolarisation is about one-third complete. The period from this point until the onset of after repolarisation is known as the relative refractory period.

What is their significance?

During the absolute refractory period, the nerve cell cannot be excited by any stimulus, no matter how strong it will be. During the relative refractory period, a stronger than normal stimulus can excite the nerve.

What is after-depolarisation? What is after-hyperpolarisation?

The slower part of the repolarisation is known as after-depolarisation. During the final recovery phase, the depolarisation process continues to have a slight overshoot beyond the resting potential. This is due to continued potassium efflux and is known as after-hyperpolarisation.

What types of neurons you are aware of? What are their characteristic features? What do you mean by saltatory conduction?

Saltatory conduction describes the conduction of an action potential along the length of a myelinated nerve through the nodes of Ranvier. Saltatory conduction in the myelinated nerves allows an increase in the speed of propagation of a nerve impulse. Table 4.4 shows types of neurons.

Table 4.4 *Classification of mammalian neurons*

Fibre Type	Function	Fibre Diameter (μ)	Conduction Speed (m/s)
Aα	Proprioception somatic motor	12–20	70–120
Aβ	Touch, pressure	5–12	30–70
Aγ	Muscle spindle motor	3–6	15–30
Aδ	Pain, temperature, touch	2–5	12–30
B	Pre-ganglionic ANS	3	3–15
C dorsal root	Pain, temperature mechanoreceptors, reflex responses	0.4–1.2	0.5–2
C sympathetic	Post-ganglionic	0.3–1.3	0.7–2.2

Pharmacology 4

Key topics: neuromuscular blocking agents, drugs acting on the gastrointestinal tract, statistics

Q1 Neuromuscular blockers

Can you classify drugs that can produce neuromuscular blockade?

Drugs that can produce neuromuscular blockade can be classified according to their mechanism of action into four types:

1 Prevention of acetylcholine synthesis (e.g. hemicholiniums).
2 Prevention of acetylcholine release (e.g. local anaesthetic agents, magnesium ions).
3 Depletion of acetylcholine stores (e.g. tetanus toxin).

4 Blockade of the acetylcholine receptor:
   (a) Depolarising blockade
      - Suxamethonium.
   (b) Non-depolarising blockade:
      - Aminosteroids – pancuronium, rocuronium, vecuronium
      - Benzylisoquinolinium esters – atracurium, mivacurium.

What are the characteristics of an ideal neuromuscular blocking agent?

- Physical:
  - Water soluble.
  - No special storage needs, long shelf-life.
  - Inexpensive.
- Pharmacokinetics:
  - Short duration of action.
  - Non-cumulative – suitable for infusion.
  - Metabolism unaffected by renal or hepatic failure.
  - Spontaneous predictable reversal.
  - Complete metabolism to inactive non-toxic metabolites.
- Pharmacodynamic:
  - Non-depolarising mode of action.
  - Rapid onset.
  - High potency.
  - No cardiovascular side effects.
  - No histamine release.
  - Safe in pregnancy and paediatrics.

What are the differentiating features between depolarising and non-depolarising blockade?

- Depolarising blockade:
  - Characterised by rapid onset with muscle fasciculation followed by relaxation.
  - Neuromuscular test stimulation shows – reduced single twitch height, reduced response to train of four – all of equal amplitude, no tetanic fade and no post-tetanic facilitation.
  - Non-competitive, cannot be antagonised by a local increase in acetylcholine levels.
- Non-depolarising blockade:
  - Relatively slower onset of action and no muscle fasciculation.
  - Neuromuscular test simulation shows –
    reduced single twitch height, reduced response to train of four, decreasing with each subsequent twitch, tetanic fade and post-tetanic facilitation.

- Competitive block can be antagonised by a local increase in acetylcholine levels and reversed with choline esterase inhibitors (neostigmine).

What is mivacurium?

Mivacurium is a non-depolarising muscle relaxant belonging to bisquaternary benzylisoquinolinium diester group.

It is a clear colourless aqueous solution with a pH of 4.5. It contains three stereoisomers: *trans–trans* (57%), *cis–trans* (36%) and *cis–cis* (6%).

How is mivacurium metabolised?

Trans–trans and *cis–trans* isomers are metabolised by plasma cholinesterase. The *cis–cis* isomer may be metabolised partly in the liver.

How is the metabolism affected in the presence of atypical or reduced plasma cholinesterase?

As with suxamethonium, in the presence of abnormal cholinesterase the duration of block is prolonged. The normal duration of action is about 20 min.

What is Hoffman degradation?

Hoffman degradation is the non-enzyme-dependent spontaneous degradation of drugs such as atracurium when exposed to body temperature and pH. In the case of atracurium the fragmentation occurs at the junction bond between the quaternary nitrogen and the central chain to form a mostly inactive metabolite, laudanosine.

How does cisatracurium differ from atracurium?

Atracurium is a mixture of 10 isomers. One of them is *cis*–cisatracurium which is isolated and marketed as cisatracurium. The cisatracurium shares most of the properties of atracurium – intermediate acting non-depolarising muscle relaxant presented as clear colourless aqueous solution to be stored in a fridge. Metabolism is similar to atracurium (Hoffman degradation and ester hydrolysis).

The most important difference is that cisatracurium causes minimal histamine release even at high doses, whereas with atracurium histamine release can cause bronchospasm and hypotension. The initial intravenous bolus dose of atracurium is 0.3–0.67 mg/kg. It is 0.15 mg/kg for cisatracurium.

Tell me about the cardiovascular side effects of non-depolarising muscle relaxants.

Non-depolarising muscle relaxants act on the post junctional nicotinic type of acetylcholine receptors, but depending upon the 'autonomic margin of safety' they can act on other acetylcholine receptors resulting in cardiovascular effects. The higher the autonomic margin of safety, lesser will be unwanted cardiovascular effects.

- Pancuronium causes vagal blockade resulting in tachycardia, increased cardiac output and hypertension. This property is often utilised in cardiac anaesthesia practice. Rocuronium also causes modest vagal blockade though not as profound as pancuronium.
- Pancuronium causes sympathetic stimulation.
- Although benzylisoquinolinium esters do not have direct cardiovascular effects, by causing histamine release they can cause hypotension and a reflex increase in heart rate. Examples include: atracurium, mivacurium.

Q2 Gastrointestinal pharmacology

Classify drugs acting on the gastrointestinal tract.

Drugs acting on the gastrointestinal tract can grossly be classified into:

- Drugs affecting secretion.
- Drugs affecting motility.

Other miscellaneous drugs such as antibiotics or drugs used in inflammatory bowel disease may be included.

What various drugs are used in the treatment of increased acidity in the upper gastrointestinal tract?

- *Drugs affecting acid secretion*: Histamine$_2$ receptor antagonists, proton pump inhibitors, prostaglandins.
- *Mucoprotective drugs*: Carbenoloxone, sucralfate, bismuth chelate.
- *Antacids*: Sodium bicarbonate, sodium citrate, aluminium hydroxide.

How does a proton pump inhibitor act?

The stomach lining contains parietal cells that secrete acid into the lumen. There is a specialised H^+/K^+ ATPase (proton pump) in these cells that catalyses the exchange of intracellular H^+ for extracellular K^+.

Proton pump inhibitors react with sulphydryl groups in the H^+/K^+ ATPase (proton pump) and cause irreversible inhibition. Acid secretion only recurs after the synthesis of new enzyme. Examples of proton pump inhibitors include omeprazole, lansoprazole.

Tell me about the role of prostaglandins in gastric acid secretion.

PGE_2 and PGI_2 inhibit gastric acid secretion. They also have mucoprotective effect by stimulating the production of mucus and bicarbonate.

Misoprostol is a synthetic PGE_2. In clinical practice it is used along with non-steroidal anti-inflammatory drugs in the prevention of ulceration.

What H_2 receptor antagonists you are aware of and how do they act?

Classification of H_2 receptor antagonists is based on their ring structure. The drugs in this group contain a five-membered ring:

- *Imidazole ring*: Cimetidine
- *Furan ring*: Ranitidine
- *Guanidinothiazole ring*: Famotidine
- *Thiazole ring*: Nizatidine

Acetylcholine and gastrin stimulate acid production indirectly by releasing histamine from paracrine cells. These paracrine cells are located close to parietal cells. Activation of parietal cells by histamine results in an increase in intracellular cAMP and secretion of acid. H_2 receptor antagonists block the action of histamine on the parietal cells and reduce acid secretion.

What are the unwanted effects of cimetidine?

- Cimetidine has an anti-androgenic effect. This may cause gynaecomastia and impotence.
- Cimetidine also inhibits cytochrome P_{450}. This can cause diminished hepatic metabolism of drugs metabolised by this enzyme system.
- Blockade of the H_2 receptor in T-lymphocytes may result in enhanced immune system activity. In post-transplant patients and in auto immune conditions this can be harmful.
- H_2 receptors are also located elsewhere in the body. In the dose used normally cimetidine has little effect on these other tissues but in susceptible patients it can act on the H_2 receptors in the atria and cause bradyarrhythmias.

What do you mean by prokinetic drugs?

Prokinetic drugs are motility stimulants that increase the contraction in stomach and enhance the emptying of stomach contents into the intestine.

What is the use of prokinetic drugs in anaesthetic practice?

In patients at risk of aspiration – full stomach, those with gastric stasis due to autonomic neuropathy as in diabetes mellitus, renal failure or patients with hiatus hernia, provided there is no distal mechanical obstruction, prokinetic drugs are used as premedication to speed the gastric emptying and to minimise the risk of aspiration.

Q3 Statistics-data

What types of statistical data are you aware of?

The two basic types of data are qualitative data and quantitative data.

- Qualitative data:
  - This type of data is non-numerical and is descriptive. This is further classified into two types, nominal and ordinal data.

    Nominal data is purely descriptive and does not have a logical order (male, female; anaesthetic technique, etc.)

    Ordinal data is descriptive, has a gradation with an order of magnitude (pain score, American Society of Anesthesiologists (ASA) grades, etc.)
- Quantitative data:
  - This type of data is numerical with equal divisions between the variables. This also includes various subtypes such as discrete data, continuous data, interval data and ratio data.

How can you describe qualitative data?

As a percentage of total number of observations. The data can be presented as frequency tables – pie diagrams or bar charts.

What about the description of quantitative data?

In quantitative data the variables represent a value on a regular continuous scale. These data are expressed as a 'central tendency' and a 'variation' around that central tendency. In normal (parametric) distribution *mean* indicates the central tendency. In non-normal (non-parametric) distribution *median* indicates the central tendency.

What did you mean by normal and non-normal distribution?

If the observed values are plotted on the x-axis and frequency plotted on the y-axis a distribution curve is produced. In a 'normal' (parametric) distribution the curve is symmetrical and is bell-shaped. In a non-normal (non-parametric) distribution the data are not normally distributed.

Tell me about the terms mean, median and mode.

These are terms used to describe the measure of 'central tendency'.

Mean is the mathematical average of values (sum of all values divided by the number of observations).

Median is the middle value, 50% of the population lie below and remaining 50% lie above the median value.

Mode is the most commonly occurring value.

In a 'normal distribution', the mean, mode and median are equal. In non-normal distribution these values vary.

What is skewing?

Skewing happens in non-normal distributions. If the mean is greater than the median, there is a positive skew and if the mean is less than the median, there is a negative skew.

What various statistical terms are used to describe the 'variability' in data?

Variability in data is used to describe the spread of data. It can be simply expressed as a *range* – that is the highest and lowest observed values. More commonly, in normal distributions, *standard deviation* (SD) is used.

Tell us more about SD. How will you measure it?

SD is the square root of variance. Variance is a measure of variation about the mean. They are measures of spread of values around the mean.

$$\text{Variance } (\sigma^2) = \Sigma(x - x')^2/N$$

Where Σ = the sum of, x = measured value, x′ = mean and N = degrees of freedom (n − 1), where n = number of observations.

1 SD includes 68% of the population; 2 SD is 95% and 3 SD is 99%.

What is standard error of the mean? How is it different from SD?

SD expresses variation about the *sample mean.* But the *confidence* with which it could be predicted that this mean of the sample represents the mean of the whole population depends on two important factors: (1) sample size and (2) variance of the sample. If the sample size is big and the variance is small then with more confidence we can claim that the sample mean represent the *population mean.* A statistical value that is derived depending on these two factors is called *standard error of the mean.* It is calculated as:

$$\text{SEM} = \text{SD}/\sqrt{N}$$

where SEM is standard error of mean, SD is standard deviation and N is the degree of freedom.

Clinical 4

Key topics: burns, carbon monoxide poisoning, Bier's block, tension pneumothorax

Q1 You have been called to the accident and emergency department to provide anaesthesia for reduction of a Colles fracture. The patient is a 68-year-old heavy smoker and drinker, who has been involved in a house fire. She has burns to her face, chest and arms

How will you assess the patient?

Airway, breathing, circulation.

Airway assessment with high index of suspicion for imminent airway obstruction.

Breathing give initially supplemental 100% oxygen. Eschars around chest can impair breathing.

Circulation with control of bleeding. Burns patients can potentially have coexisting injuries that require immediate attention.

Assessment and management of the patient should go hand with hand. After completing the primary survey and stabilising the vital signs secondary survey should be carried out to identify other injuries.

The extent of burns is classically determined by 'rule of nines'.

Once stabilised, if the patient is coming to theatre for a surgical intervention a comprehensive anaesthetic history including previous surgery and anaesthesia, past medical history, drugs and allergies, nil by mouth status, etc. should be elicited.

Discuss her airway assessment in more detail.

Her airway assessment comprises two main issues:

- Assessment of airway in presence of burns.
- General assessment of airway for identifying anticipated difficult intubation.

Airway in burns: Burns to face and neck are an imminent threat for airway obstruction. Features of inhalation injury – carbonaceous soot in sputum, singeing of nasal hair, hoarseness of voice should be sought. These patients often need early intubation as delay can lead to severe airway oedema and make subsequent airway management difficult.

General assessment of the airway:

For details see SOE 8, Clinical 8.

What are the indications for intubation? Will you use suxamethonium? What other precautions would you take?

Indications are:

- Facial burns.
- Suspicion of inhalation injury.
- Plan to transfer the patient.

Due to the proliferation of extra-junctional receptors a severe hyperkalaemic response following suxamethonium can happen from 1 to 10 weeks following burns. In the early stages of resuscitation suxamethonium can safely be used.

For intubation, an uncut endotracheal tube must be used as subsequent facial oedema can be severe enough to 'engulf' a tube.

What fluid requirements will the patient have? What fluid would you give, when would you give it, and why?

There is a tendency for generalised capillary leakiness and increased third space fluid loss in burns. Various fluid regimens are available. The Parkland formula is often used, which is 4 ml/kg/% total body surface area burnt. Half of the calculated volume should be given in first 8 h (calculated from the time of burns) and the remaining over next 16 h. This is in addition to the normal maintenance fluid of 1–2 ml/kg/h.

Burns patients can often have associated injuries and concealed bleeding which need to be appropriately addressed. These formulae are for guidance only and the actual fluid management should be determined by the clinical situation and frequent assessment of hydration status with parameters such as urine output.

What about the pain management in burns?

Burns produce excruciating pain. Although the myth is that total thickness burns are not very painful due to loss of sensation, the reality is that it is equally or even more painful due to inflammation of adjacent tissues.

The various analgesic options available include:

- Intravenous opioid analgesics (e.g. morphine, patient-controlled analgesia).
- Ketamine.
- Inhalation of entonox, particularly for changing dressings.

Discuss the significance of SpO_2 in burns. What are the shortcomings and how would you over come them?

Pulse oximetry readings can be misleading in the burns due to the presence of carboxyhaemoglobin in blood that tends to show a saturation nearing 100%. Currently available pulse oximeters have only two diodes and hence cannot detect abnormal haemoglobins. Oximeters using a range of wavelengths to measure all forms of haemoglobins are available and can be used for assessing carboxyhaemoglobin levels.

What are the effects of carbon monoxide poisoning?

Carbon monoxide affects oxygen transport and utilisation. It has 200 times more affinity for haemoglobin than oxygen. Therefore:

- A reduced amount of haemoglobin is available for oxygen transport.
- A left shift of the oxygen dissociation curve impairs oxygen delivery to tissues.
- Carbon monoxide binds to cytochrome oxidase and impairs tissue oxygen utilisation.
- There is direct cardio-vascular depression.

How can you treat carbon monoxide poisoning?

100% oxygen decreases the half-life of carboxyhaemoglobin from about 4–1 h. Hyperbaric oxygen is useful in severe poisoning causing coma, persistent acidosis, myocardial ischaemia, etc. Hyperbaric oxygen can reduce the half-life to less than ½h.

How would you anaesthetise for reduction of Colles fracture in this lady?

After initial resuscitation and stabilisation, the options available include general anaesthesia and regional anaesthesia.

Tell me more about the available regional anaesthesia techniques.

- Brachial plexus nerve block.
- Intravenous regional anaesthesia (Bier's block).
- Haematoma block (local infiltration).

Q2 Critical incident: pneumothorax

What would you do if an anaesthetised patient suddenly became hard to ventilate?

Look for the cause which can be anywhere between the patient and the machine. Briefly check for obvious causes, like an obvious kink in the circuit or wearing off of muscle relaxant. Call for senior help, work back from patient to machine in a logical manner. Consider changing onto portable cylinder and Waters circuit if all else fails – remembering recent reports of plastic debris within circuit components.

What are the possible causes for this scenario?

- Wearing off of muscle relaxant.
- Bronchospasm.
- Anaphylaxis.
- Tension pneumothorax.
- Endobronchial intubation, obstruction to the tube with secretions, cuff herniation.
- Kinked endotracheal tube or obstruction to the circuit.

- Ventilator malfunction.
- Circuit obstructions.

What will be the findings in tension pneumothorax?

- *Inspection*: Cyanosis, diminished movement of affected chest, tracheal shift
- *Auscultation*: Diminished air entry on affected side
- *Percussion*: Hyper-resonance
- *Monitoring*: Desaturation, tachycardia, hypotension, distorted end tidal CO_2 ($ETCO_2$)
- *Investigation*: Chest X-ray can confirm the diagnosis but *tension pneumothorax is a medical emergency that should be diagnosed clinically.*

How will you treat tension pneumothorax?

- 100% oxygen.
- Immediate decompression of the tension with a wide bore cannula through second intercostal space, midclavicular line.
- Haemodynamic support with fluids.
- Definitive management is with a proper intercostal drain in the fifth intercostal space, midaxillary line.

Q3 What aids are available for difficult intubation?

These can be listed in order of priority into:

- *Gum elastic bougie*: This simple device is probably the single most important aid. It is a 60-cm-long introducer, with a smooth angled tip at the end. The bougie is made from braided polyester with a resin coat which provides both the necessary stiffness and flexibility to enable it to be passed into the larynx (disposable versions are now advocated). It may be bent prior to insertion to aid placement. The device is especially useful in cases where the glottic opening cannot be visualised. In this situation correct placement may be confirmed by the detection of clicks as the introducer is gently passed down into the trachea. The tracheal tube can then be slid over the bougie into the trachea with a 90° anti-clockwise rotation to facilitate passage through the laryngeal inlet.
- *Stylet*: A precurved malleable stylet can be placed within an endotracheal tube to enable the tube to be curved and thus aid placement of the tube especially when the larynx is anteriorly situated. The stylet should on no account be allowed to protrude beyond the tip of the endotracheal tube, as this may cause trauma to the larynx.
- *Lightwand*: A lightwand uses the principle of transillumination of the neck when a light is passed into the trachea. In this situation a distinct glow can be seen below the thyroid cartilage which is not apparent when the light is placed in the oesophagus.

- *Alternative laryngoscope blades*: Several different laryngoscope blades are now available.

  The standard Macintosh laryngoscope has a relatively short curved blade designed to rest in the vallecula and lift the epiglottis. Other useful designs include:
  - *Miller*: Straight bladed laryngoscope with a slight curve at the tip. The blade is longer, narrower and smaller at the tip and is designed to trap and lift the epiglottis.
  - *McCoy*: The McCoy levering laryngoscope has a hinged blade tip controlled by a spring-loaded lever on the handle of the laryngoscope which allows elevation of the epiglottis without the use of excessive forces on the pharyngeal tissues.
  - *Bullard*: The Bullard laryngoscope is a rigid bladed indirect fibreoptic laryngoscope with a shape designed to match the airway. A fibreoptic bundle passes along the posterior aspect of the blade allowing excellent visualisation of the larynx. Intubation can be achieved using an attached intubating stylet with preloaded endotracheal tube.
  - *Prism*: The Huffman prism is one example of a laryngoscope using refraction to aid visualisation of the larynx. It employs a modification of the Macintosh blade whereby a block of transparent plastic in a prism shape is attached to the proximal end of the blade. The ends of the prism are polished to provide optically flat surfaces, the nearest to the eye being cut at 90° to the line of vision and the distal surface at 30°. The net result to the view obtained is a refraction of approximately 30°.
  - *Polio*: The Polio blade was originally designed to enable patients in an iron lung to be ventilated. In the UK the 'polio blade' is actually a 90° adapter located between the handle and blade of a standard Macintosh laryngoscope. It allows the easier introduction of the blade in situations where the chest gets in the way of the handle.
- *Laryngeal mask airway*: The laryngeal mask airway (LMA) is a useful means of airway control in difficult and failed intubations. The intubating LMA allows an endotracheal tube to be placed blindly. There are now numerous supraglottic airway devices which may or may not help oxygenation in the early management of difficult intubation.
- *Blind nasal intubation*: If skilled enough a blind nasal intubation is possible. A nasotracheal tube is passed through the nose with the head extended at the atlanto-axial joint. The tip of the tube, if kept in the midline, will usually impact anteriorly and flexion of the head will allow advancement of the tube into the larynx.

What do you understand by retrograde intubation?

Retrogade intubation involves the passage of a catheter through a crico-thyroid incision upwards so as to protrude at the mouth. It is then possible to use the catheter to railroad an endotracheal tube into the larynx. The technique may be carried out under local or general anaesthesia but it has complications.

What are the possible complications?

Complications of retrograde intubation include the following:

- Bleeding.
- Perforation of posterior wall of trachea with needle.
- Subcutaneous emphysema of neck.
- Pneumothorax.
- Infection at puncture site.

Physics, clinical measurement and safety 4

Key topics: flow, gas and gas laws, electrical safety

Q1 Flow

Tell me what intravenous (IV) cannula would you like to insert in 60-year-old male posted for laparotomy? Why?

A minimum size is at least a 14- or 16-G cannula for IV infusion. Laparotomy involves huge fluid shifts and rapid transfusion of fluids for replacement and resuscitation is indicated, therefore the cannula must permit high flow rates.

What does G stand for?

G refers to gauge. When describing the calibre of cannulae or needles the unit SWG (Standard Wire Gauge) is used. The smaller the number, the bigger will be the size of the cannula.

What is French gauge?

French gauge is used to measure nasogastric tubes, double-lumen tubes. This value represents circumference (internal diameter $\times$ π). The bigger the number, the bigger will be the size of the tube.

Can you tell me how much flow can occur through these IV cannulae? Shows picture of orange, grey, white, green, pink and blue venflon type cannulae.

- *Orange*: 14G = 250–360 ml/min
- *Grey*: 16G = 130–220 ml/min
- *White*: 17G = 100–140 ml/min

- *Green*: 18G = 75–120 ml/min
- *Pink*: 20G = 40–80 ml/min
- *Blue*: 22G = 20–40 ml/min

This is a common colour coding but it can vary with manufacturers. The flows described are in certain standardised conditions where distilled water at a temperature of 22°C is used. This runs under a pressure of 10 kPa through a tubing of 4 mm internal diameter and 110 cm length.

If you double the diameter of the IV cannula, by what factor will the flow increase? Why?

The flow increases by a factor of 16. This is defined by the Hagen–Poiseuille formula, Flow = $\pi r^4 \Delta P/8\eta l$. So if radius is doubled flow increases by 2^4 times, which is 16.

What happens to the blood flow in polycythaemia?

In polycythaemia viscosity is increased and so flow is decreased.

What do you mean by viscosity?

Viscosity is a measure of the frictional forces acting between the layers of the fluid as it flows along the tube. The unit is 'pascal seconds'.

What is the difference between laminar and turbulent flow?

In laminar flow fluid moves in a steady manner and there are no eddies or turbulence. During laminar flow there is a linear relationship between flow and pressure ($P/Q = R$, P is pressure, Q is flow and R is the resistance in the tube). Laminar flow occurs in smoother tubes at lower flow rates.

These characteristics are lost in turbulent flow. The fluid flows with eddies and turbulence. There is increased resistance to the flow and the relation between pressure (P) and flow (Q) does not exist any longer.

The transition between laminar and turbulent occurs when Reynold's number exceeds 2000.

$$R = v\rho d/\eta$$

(v is velocity, ρ is density, d is diameter and η is viscosity).

Can you name some implications of turbulent and laminar flow in your anaesthetic practice?

- Avoiding right angled connectors and sharp bends in the breathing system to avoid turbulence.
- Airway tumour causes turbulent flow. Heliox can reduce the density and increases the flow.

- In flow meters during lower flow rates laminar flow is maintained (and hence viscosity is important). At higher flow rate turbulent flow predominates (and hence density is important).
- Turbulent flow in blood vessels cause bruits and through valves causes murmurs.
- Choosing appropriate calibre infusion sets and IV cannula for fluid administration. When denser fluids like colloids are administered under pressure through thin and lengthier tubing turbulence occurs and flow becomes poorer.

What is the Venturi principle?

The Venturi principle is entrainment of a fluid through a side arm into an area of low pressure caused by a constriction in the tube.

Why does this happen?

Energy is neither created nor destroyed but is converted from one form to another. When the fluid flows through a constriction in the tube the pressure drops (potential energy). There is considerable increase in the fluid velocity (kinetic energy). The total energy remains constant.

What is entrainment ratio?

$$\text{Entrainment ratio} = \text{entrained flow}/\text{driving flow}$$

Give some clinical applications of the Venturi principle.

Venturi principle is applied in oxygen delivery devices, Sanders injector, jet ventilators, suction devices, humidifiers and nebulisers.

What is the Coanda effect?

The Coanda effect describes channelling of flow. There is a fall in pressure and increase in the speed of the fluid when it passes through a narrowed tube. Unlike the classical Venturi effect if there are no vents in the side wall to entrain other fluids but rather a solid surface, then the fluid stream is held against the wall of the tube in the region of low pressure. If this tube divides into 'Y'-shaped two outlets, the flow does not split into two streams but flows through only one limb of the 'Y'.

In the body this effect can be explained in the behaviour of blood flows beyond a constriction as in coronary artery disease and in maldistribution of gas flow in chronic obstructive airway diseases. This effect is also used in 'fluid logic' ventilators.

Q2 Gas laws

Can you tell me the differences between solid, liquid and gas?

- *Solid*: Attractive forces (van der Waals forces) bind the molecules together, so molecules oscillate around a fixed point but are tightly bound together.

- *Liquid*: Intermolecular forces are weak but still strong enough to give a definite volume and surface tension.
- *Gas*: Molecules are separated from each other and they are free to move.

What is the effect of increasing temperature on kinetic energy?

Kinetic energy is increased and the molecules move apart. Solid such as ice can turn into liquid, then in to gas or vapour.

Can you define critical temperature?

It is the temperature above which a gas cannot be liquefied, no matter how much pressure is applied.

Can you define critical pressure?

It is the pressure needed to liquefy the gas at critical temperature.

What is the difference between a gas and vapour ?

Gas is the substance above the critical temperature. Gaseous substance below the critical temperature is called vapour. This means gas cannot be liquefied but vapour can be liquefied by applying enough pressure.

Can you explain this graph concerning nitrous oxide?

This is a graph of isotherms for nitrous oxide with volume on the x-axis and pressure on the y-axis. The relation between pressure and volume is shown at various temperatures.

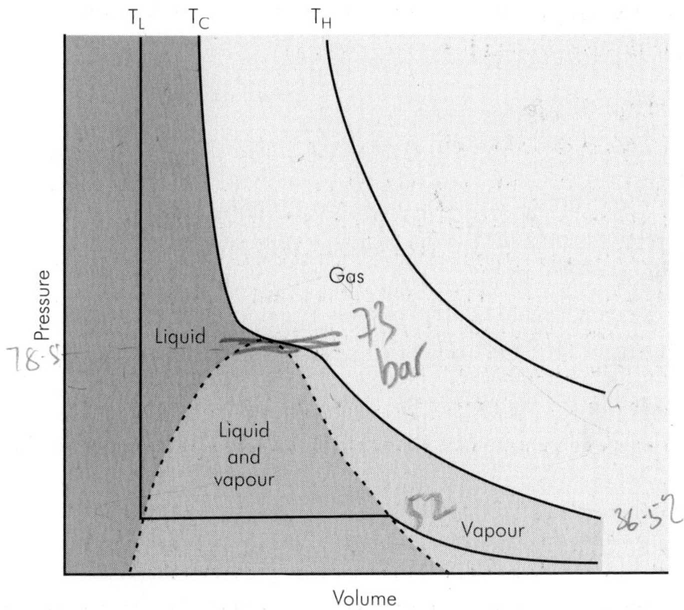

Figure 4.4 *Isotherms of nitrous oxide*

- *Line at T_H* – This is above critical temperature. At this temperature nitrous oxide exists only as gas. It cannot be liquefied at this temperature. Reducing the volume will result in increasing the pressure, producing a rectangular hyperbola.
- *Line at T_C* – This is at the critical temperature of nitrous oxide which is 36.5°C. Critical pressure of nitrous oxide is 73 bar which can liquefy nitrous oxide at this temperature. As liquid is relatively incompressible, any reduction in volume will cause a sharp rise in pressure producing a straight line above this pressure.
- *Line at T_L* – This is below critical temperature. At a pressure of 52 bar some of the nitrous oxide liquefies. At this temperature it is present in both liquid and gas form. Further decrease in volume causes more gas to liquefy and pressure remains unaltered, hence horizontal line is produced. This is the working pressure in the nitrous oxide cylinder.

What is Boyle's law?
At constant temperature the volume of a fixed mass of a perfect gas is inversely proportional to the pressure.

Can you tell me a clinical application of Boyle's law?
It can be applied to calculate available oxygen from an oxygen cylinder.

If the cylinder volume is 10 l and the gauge pressure is 137 bar, if you use oxygen at a rate of 10 l/min how long does it last?
Assume the temperature remains the same throughout. If the gauge pressure is 137 bar then the absolute pressure is 138 bar (gauge pressure + atmospheric pressure).

By Boyle's law

$$P_1 V_1 = P_2 V_2$$

Where P_1 is the cylinder pressure, V_1 is the cylinder volume, P_2 is the ambient (atmospheric) pressure and V_2 is the available volume of oxygen.

Therefore, $138 \times 10 = 1 \times V_2$.

This cylinder can provide 1380 l of oxygen. The last 10 l of oxygen within the cylinder cannot be used. So, when used at 10 l/min it will last for 137 min.

What is Charles law?
At constant pressure volume of a given gas is directly proportional to the absolute temperature.

Can you write down the universal gas law?

$$PV = nRT$$

(n is number of moles of a gas, R is the universal gas constant and T is temperature).

How many molecules are there in 32 g of oxygen?

Molecular weight of oxygen is 32. 32 g of oxygen is therefore one mole and according to Avogadro's number it will contain 6.023×10^{23} molecules.

What is Avogadro's hypothesis?

Equal volumes of all gases under same conditions of temperature and pressure contain the same number of molecules. At STP 1 g molecular weight of a gas occupies a volume of 22.4 l (STP: **S**tandard **T**emperature: 0°C, **P**ressure: 101.3 kPa).

Can you tell me the volume of vapour that can be obtained from 10 ml of isoflurane at STP?

- The molecular weight of isoflurane is 185. Therefore 185 g of isoflurane will produce 22.4 l of vapour at STP. 10 g will produce 1210 ml of vapour.
- As the density of isoflurane is 1.5, 10 ml of isoflurane weighs 15 g.
- By calculation, 10 ml will produce 1815 ml of vapour (1210×1.5).

Q3 Electrical safety and diathermy

What is the frequency and voltage of the mains electricity in UK?

50 Hz and 240 V.

What is Ohm's law?

$I = V/R$, I is current flow, V is potential difference or voltage and R the resistance (*analogue*: $Q = P/R$, Q is flow, P is pressure difference and R is resistance).

What is a conductor?

Materials in which electrons are loosely bound and can move through the material under the influence of an electric potential are called conductors (metals, carbon, saline, body fluids).

What are insulators and semiconductors?

In insulators electrons are firmly bound and are not able to move. Insulators do not conduct electricity.

In semiconductors electrons are bound less firmly than in an insulator. In normal conditions they do not conduct electricity. But by applying energy semiconductors can be converted in to conductors. This property is used in thermistor, transistors, etc.

In a thermistor heat energy (i.e. increased temperature) converts a semiconductor into a conductor.

What is alternating current? How does it differ from direct current?

In alternating current (AC) flow of electrons is first in one direction and then in the opposite direction. In direct current (DC) flow of electrons is only in one direction.

What is diathermy? How does it work?

Diathermy is a piece of electrical equipment that employs high-frequency AC to cut and coagulate tissues. When high-frequency current passes through a small area the current density (current per unit area) is sufficient to cut or coagulate the tissues.

What are the different types of diathermy?

It can be monopolar or bipolar. In monopolar diathermy there is one active electrode to deliver the current. The current leaves the body from the neutral plate.

Bipolar diathermy does not need a neutral plate. There are two electrodes designed like specialised forceps, one to deliver the current and other to complete the circuit. Usually bipolar diathermy requires lower power output and has applications in areas such as paediatric and neurosurgery.

What are the problems encountered when using diathermy?

- If the neutral plate is totally disconnected then current will flow through the patient and get earthed through any conducting objects touching the patient. This can cause burns. If the neutral plate is poorly adhered to the patient then current leaves the patient through a smaller area due to poorer contact of the pad. The current density (current/area) is increased leading to the risk of burns.
- Fires and explosion. Avoidance of inflammable anaesthetic vapours has reduced the risks, but alcohol based cleansing and the bowel gases with inflammable properties can be ignited with diathermy.
- Pacemaker malfunction.

What safety feature within the diathermy machine prevents electrocution?

- An isolating capacitor in the diathermy circuit provides high impedance for the low frequency current, but very low impedance for the high frequency diathermy current.
- Use of a floating circuit.

What is a floating circuit?

A floating circuit, also called an isolated circuit, consists of two coils insulated from each other. Current flow in the primary coil induces current in the secondary coil (patient coil). Primary coil is earthed. Secondary coil is floating (not earthed). Thus the patient who is in contact with the secondary coil is not directly earthed but is in 'floating circuit'.

What factors determine the extent of injury following an electric shock?

The amount of current, current density, current pathway, duration of exposure, frequency of current and the type of current (DC or AC) determine the extent of injury. AC at 50 Hz is the most dangerous. Frequencies more than 1 kHz are generally safer.

What are the physiological effects at different current levels in AC mains shock?

- At 0–5 mA it gives tingling sensation.
- Between 5 and 10 mA it causes pain.
- From 10 to 50 mA the pain can be quite severe; muscle spasm will accompany.
- 50–100 mA is sufficient to cause respiratory muscle spasm, ventricular fibrillation and myocardial failure.

How can we prevent electrocution in theatre?

- Proper maintenance of electrical equipment.
- Precautions to ensure patient is not in contact with the earthed equipment.
- Measures to avoid building up of static electricity – antistatic shoes with high impedance, flooring, etc.
- Equipment design.
- Isolated circuits and circuit breakers.

Tell me more about the equipment design.

Equipment is classified based on the degree of protection, or based on the maximum permissible leakage current:

- *Classification according to their protection*:
  - Class I: Earthed, fuse incorporated into the system.
  - Class II: Double or reinforced insulation, earth wire is not required.
  - Class III: Internally powered by battery.
- *Classification according to maximum permissible leakage currents*:
  - Type B: Maximum leakage current must not exceed 100 μA. These can come into contact with body.
  - Type BF: Floating/isolated circuit consisting of isolating transformer, two coils.
  - Type CF: Maximum leakage is less than 10 μA (e.g. pulmonary artery catheters). These are suitable for direct cardiac connection.

What is microshock?

AC mains electricity can produce small currents in the body by inductive coupling and capacitive coupling. Such currents are called leakage currents and generally will not cause gross electric shock, although in certain circumstances they can lead to a potential danger called microshock.

Even a current as small as 150 μA when passing through a very small area in myocardium can result in high current density (current per unit area) resulting in ventricular fibrillation. This can occur with any equipment that comes into direct contact with the wall of the heart – such as a faulty intracardiac catheter. This phenomenon is called microshock.

SOE 5

Physiology 5

Key topics: pacemaker cell, cell membrane, spinal cord tracts

Q1 Pacemaker cells

Can you tell me about the origin and conduction of the cardiac impulse?

It originates at the sino-atrial (SA) node, from there it is conducted to the atrio-ventricular (AV) node and from there it spreads to the myocardium through the bundle of His, bundle branches and Purkinje fibres.

How does the impulse pass from SA node to AV node?

There are three bundles of atrial fibres that connect the SA node to the AV node; they are anterior (Bachmann), middle (Wenckebach) and posterior (Thorel) tracts.

What is special about the action potential of the SA node?

The SA node has modified myocardial cells that have a special property known as a pacemaker potential where during the repolarisation phase, the membrane potential declines to the threshold level and spontaneously triggers the next impulse. This is called *automaticity* of pacemaker cells and it depends on the leakage of sodium into the cell in the Phase 4 of action potential causing spontaneous depolarisation. Pacemaker cells also maintain a regular discharge rate, a property described as *rhythmicity*.

Can you draw a diagram to describe the pacemaker action potential and explain the reasons for those changes?

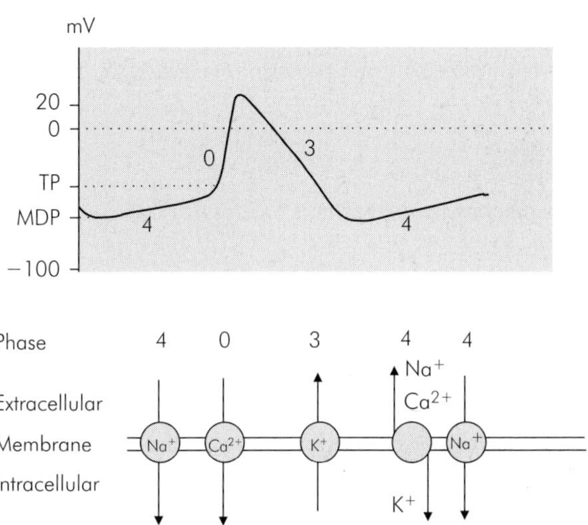

Figure 5.1 *Pacemaker action potential*

The pacemaker action potential is described as a *slow response action potential* that has three distinctive phases:

1 *Phase 4*: resting stage
2 *Phase 0*: rapid depolarisation
3 *Phase 3*: repolarisation

Phase 4: Unlike rest of myocardium, pacemaker cells do not have a stable resting membrane potential (RMP). Owing to increased membrane permeability to sodium and calcium ions they tend to demonstrate '*spontaneous diastolic depolarisation*'. When the membrane potential changes from maximum diastolic depolarisation (MDP) of −60 mV to a threshold potential (TP) of −40 mV Phase 0 occurs.

Phase 0: At TP there is influx of calcium ions through the T-type calcium channels leading to rapid depolarisation.

Phase 3: Potassium ion efflux results in repolarisation.

How does this pacemaker action potential differ from the action potential of cardiac muscle?

- Phase 4 membrane potential is less negative in pacemaker cells (MDP of −60 mV against RMP of −90 mV in myocardial cells).
- Less negative TP.
- Spontaneous diastolic depolarisation due to leakiness of membranes of pacemaker cells.

- Phase 0 in pacemaker cells is due to 'slower calcium ion influx' rather than 'fast sodium ion influx' in myocytes. Therefore less steep slope.
- Pacemaker action potential repolarisation is effectively a single phase (Phase 3) as there is no Phase 1 (early rapid repolarisation) and very brief Phase 2 (plateau). Whereas myocyte repolarisation has distinctive Phases 1, 2 and 3.

Q2 Cell membranes

Can you name the mechanisms by which solutes are transported across the capillary endothelium?

- *Filtration*: hydrostatic pressure forces the fluid out of the capillary (both solute and solvent), for example in glomerular filtration.
- *Diffusion*: passive movement across a concentration gradient.
- *Transcytosis*: active transfer of substance by endocytosis from the capillary lumen and then by exocytosis out of the endothelial cells.

What is the Gibbs–Donnan effect?

The Gibbs–Donnan effect describes the effect of a non-diffusible charged particle on one side of the membrane on the distribution of the other charged particles that can freely diffuse across the membrane. As a result, in equilibrium, there is a fixed ratio between the concentrations of the diffusible ions on either side of the membrane:

$$[Na^+]_A \times [Cl^-]_A = [Na^+]_B \times [Cl^-]_B$$

where subscripts A and B are two compartments separated by a semipermeable membrane.

For example, proteins are negatively charged and are not freely diffusible across the membranes. These negative charges hold the Na^+ back on one side of the compartment to maintain electrical neutrality. For any movement across membrane there are two major determinants – electrical gradient and chemical gradient. Therefore, the chemical gradient of Na^+ across the membrane will then redistribute Na^+ between the compartments until equilibrium is reached. Cl^- follows Na^+ to preserve electrical neutrality.

The Gibbs–Donnan effect gives rise to:

- An unequal distribution of Na^+ and Cl^- ions between the intravascular and interstitial compartments.
- Higher sodium content in the protein containing plasma compartment and higher Cl^- concentration in the interstitial compartment.
- A small electrical potential difference across the membrane. The magnitude of this potential is calculated using the Nernst equation.

Tell me more about the Nernst equation.

The Nernst equation is used in calculating the potential difference on either side of a biological membrane. This relies on the ratio of the diffusible ion concentrations on either side of the membrane concerned. For example, across the capillary wall, the potential is:

$$RT/FZ_{Na^+} \times \log_e [Na^+]_{INT}/[Na^+]_C$$

where R is the gas constant; T is the absolute temperature; F is the Faraday constant (no. of coulombs per mole of charge); Z is the valency; INT is the interstitium; C is the capillary.

In case of capillaries this potential difference is about −3 mV.

What is osmosis?

When two compartments containing solutes of different concentrations are separated by a semipermeable membrane, a net movement of water occurs across the semipermeable membrane due to diffusion from the area of lower concentration of solute to the area of higher concentration of solute. This property is called osmosis.

What is osmotic pressure?

The movement of water into a compartment with a higher concentration of solute increases the volume of the compartment with or without increase in its pressure. This movement of water can be opposed by an increase in the pressure in that compartment. The pressure required to oppose the net movement of water into a solution is described as osmotic pressure. It is therefore 'the pressure required to prevent osmosis'.

What is the difference between osmolarity and osmolality?

The concentration of solute particles in solution is expressed in osmoles (One osmole is the amount of solute that exerts an osmotic pressure of 1 atm when placed in 22.4 l of solution at 0°C).

Osmolarity is concentration of solution expressed in osmoles of solute per litre of solution (solute + water).

Osmolality is concentration of solution expressed as osmoles of solute per kilogram solvent (water alone).

As the osmolality is independent of temperature, and independent of the volume taken up by the solutes within the solution, it is a preferred expression in most physiological applications.

Q3 Spinal cord tracts

Describe the anatomy of the spinal cord.

The spinal cord is the continuation of the medulla and begins at the level of foramen magnum and ends at the level of first or second lumbar vertebrae to continue as the conus medullaris.

The cord comprises a central canal containing cerebrospinal fluid (CSF), surrounded by grey matter with anterior and posterior horns, which is surrounded by white matter containing the ascending and descending tracts. It is covered by three membranes: dura mater, arachnoid and pia mater.

What is the arterial blood supply to the spinal cord?

The blood supply is from a single anterior spinal artery and two posterior spinal arteries. The single anterior spinal artery lies in the anterior median sulcus and is formed at the level of foramen magnum by the union of two vertebral arteries. It supplies the anterior two-thirds of the cord.

The posterior one-third of the cord is supplied by the paired small posterior spinal arteries, derived from the posterior inferior cerebellar arteries. There are additional supplies from various radicular branches from cervical, intercostal and lumbar arteries. There is also a direct supply from the aorta called the artery of Adamkiewicz, at the level of about T_{11} to L_3 which is crucial in supplying the lower two-thirds of spinal cord.

Can you draw me the diagram of the transverse section of spinal cord and name the various ascending and descending tracts?

The cord has slight grooves in the midline on both anterior and posterior surfaces. These are known as the anterior median fissure and posterior median sulcus respectively. In the centre there is a central canal that contains CSF. The central canal is surrounded by an area of grey matter. Grey matter has two anterior and two posterior horns. Grey matter is in turn surrounded by the white matter which contains the ascending and descending tracts.

What are the effects of acute spinal cord injury on various systems?

Complete transaction:

- Spinal shock occurs immediately after injury and lasts between a few hours and 3–6 weeks. Flaccid paralysis below the level of injury, loss of vascular tone and vasopressor reflex, paralytic ileus and visceral and somatic sensory loss is common.
- A lesion at T_7 or above causes alteration in respiratory function due to a decrease in vital capacity, expiratory reserve volume and FEV_1.
- Loss of sympathetic nervous system activity from T_1–L_2 leads to vasodilation, blood pooling, orthostatic hypotension and bradycardia.
- A C_6 lesion leaves the diaphragm intact. Intercostal muscle paralysis results in diminished effectiveness to cough.

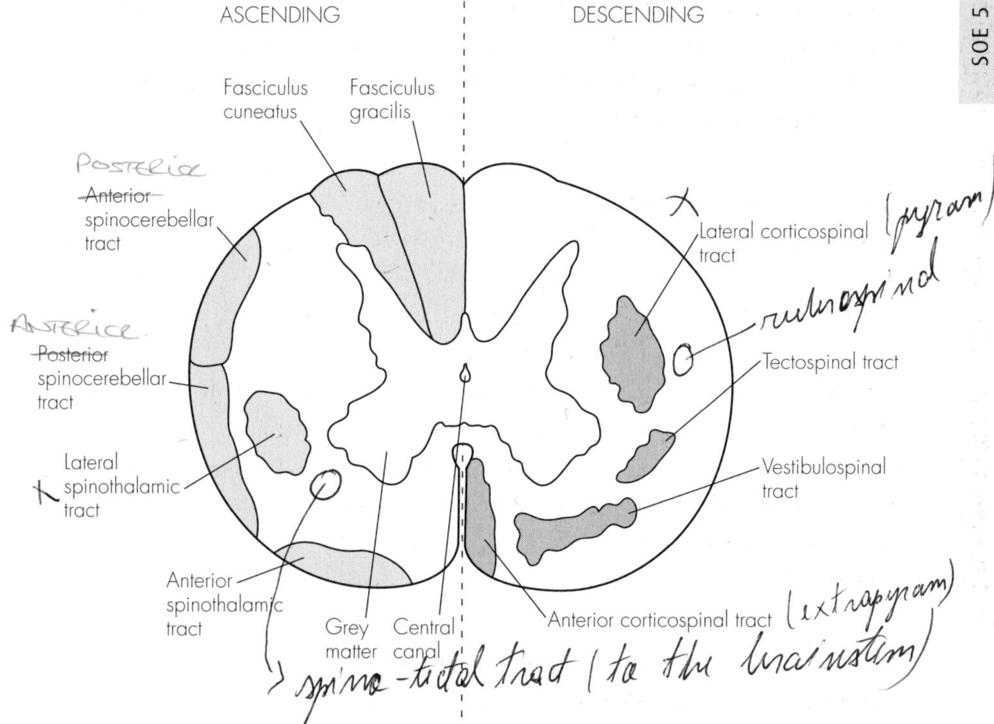

Figure 5.2 *Tracts of the spinal cord*

- Lesion at C_4 or above results in diaphragmatic paralysis and grossly impaired ventilation.
- Gastric paralysis and paralytic ileus leads to abdominal distension which also impairs ventilation. There is an increased risk of aspiration due to increased secretion (paralysed sympathetic nervous system), gastric dilation and ineffective cough.
- Thermoregulation is impaired.
- Respiratory acidosis (hypoventilation), metabolic alkalosis and hypokalaemia (vomiting and gastric suctioning) ensues eventually.

Hemisection of spinal cord:

This is also called Brown Sequard syndrome. There is loss of muscle motor activity, touch, pressure and proprioception senses on the same side. The temperature and pain sensation from the opposite side are affected. This is because of involvement of pyramidal tract and posterior columns on the ipsilateral side and inclusion of the spinothalamic tract that has crossed over from the opposite side carrying temperature and pain sensation.

Pharmacology 5

Key topics: nitrous oxide, pharmacokinetics (V_d and TIVA), hypoglycaemic drugs

Q1 Nitrous oxide

Tell me about the physical properties of nitrous oxide.

Nitrous oxide has a molecular weight of 44. Its boiling point is −88°C with a saturated vapour pressure of 5300 kPa. The critical temperature and the critical pressure are 36.5°C and 72.6 bar, respectively. It is supplied in cylinders as liquid under a pressure of 44 bar. When inhaled, the blood/gas partition coefficient is 0.47.

What is the minimum alveolar concentration (MAC) of nitrous oxide?

Between 101 and 105.

How is nitrous oxide manufactured?

Nitrous oxide is manufactured by heating ammonium nitrate between 240°C and 270°C. Impurities such as ammonia, carbon monoxide, chlorine, higher oxides of nitrogen and water vapour are removed by treating with potassium permanganate solution and sulphuric acid.

What properties of nitrous oxide have favoured its clinical use?

- Due to low blood gas solubility there is rapid equilibration of the brain concentration with the inhaled concentration.
- Although by itself it is not very potent, when combined with other inhalation and intravenous agents it forms a useful adjunct, reducing the MAC of other volatile agents.
- It has an analgesic effect.
- Minimal adverse effects at clinically used concentrations, non-irritant.
- Speeds up inhalation induction by the concentration effect (for an agent with low blood gas solubility) and second gas effect (for an agent with high blood gas solubility). Nitrous oxide diffuses 14 times faster than oxygen, thereby relatively increasing the alveolar concentration of an agent with a high blood gas solubility.

How can you explain the analgesic effect of nitrous oxide?

Nitrous oxide acts on the periaqueductal grey (PAG) area of the midbrain, to release neuropeptides (endorphins and encephalins) which stimulate descending inhibitory pathways thereby modulating neurotransmission at the dorsal horn of spinal cord.

What are the disadvantages of nitrous oxide?

- Nitrous oxide diffuses 25 times faster than nitrogen and will therefore rapidly diffuse into closed spaces.
- Postoperative nausea and vomiting may be increased.
- In the presence of pulmonary hypertension, it increases the pulmonary vascular resistance.
- On prolonged exposure nitrous oxide can interact with vitamin B_{12} and inhibit deoxyribonucleic acid (DNA) synthesis causing megaloblastic anaemia, fetotoxic effects and neuropathy.

Q2 Pharmacokinetics (V_d and TIVA)

Define volume of distribution.

Volume of distribution represents the apparent volume available in the body for the distribution of the drug. It does not necessarily correspond to anatomical or physiological tissue compartments.

What are the factors that affect volume of distribution of a drug?

- Partition coefficient of the drug.
- Regional blood flow to the tissues.
- Degree of plasma protein binding.
- Degree of tissue protein binding.

Drugs that are highly lipid soluble, such as digoxin, have a very high volume of distribution (500 l). Drugs which are lipid insoluble, such as neuromuscular blockers, remain in the blood and therefore have a low volume of distribution.

How volume of distribution is measured?

It is not measured clinically because it is not an actual volume. Volume of distribution (V_d) is the amount of drug in the body divided by the concentration in the blood.

V_d = dose/concentration of drug. It can be extrapolated from a concentration time curve after intravenous administration.

What is elimination half-life?

Elimination half-life (t½) is the time taken for plasma concentration (Cp) to reduce by 50%. After four half-lives, elimination is 94% complete.

What is context sensitive half-life?

In relation to intravenous infusion, it is the time required for the drug concentration to fall by half at the end of a period of infusion designed to maintain a constant concentration. 'Context' is the duration of infusion.

What is the significance of Cp and effect site concentration (Ce)?

- Cp: drug concentration in the plasma.
- Ce: drug concentration at the site of effect. For intravenous anaesthetic agents the site of effect is brain.
- At induction Cp > Ce, at maintenance Cp = Ce, at emergence Ce > Cp.

Can you measure Ce of propofol?

No. Using mathematical equations modern infusion devices gives a value for possible effective site concentration. These values are derived from animal models. The concentration of propofol in the cerebral venous system closely relates to brain concentration. To be accurate, one should measure the concentration at brain tissue or more precisely at receptors.

Define Cp50. What is the use of knowing Cp50?

It is the Cp at which motor response in 50% of unpremedicated patients to skin incision is prevented. This value is used to compare the potency of drugs.

What is total intravenous anaesthesia (TIVA) and what are its advantages?

TIVA stands for total intravenous anaesthesia in which only the intravenous route is used for providing anaesthesia.

The advantages of TIVA include avoidance of problems associated with use of inhaled anaesthetic agents such as:

- Production of fluoride ions associated with some newer volatile agents.
- Distension of air-filled spaces within the patient.
- Postoperative diffusion hypoxaemia.
- Ponv.
- Occupational exposure to inhalation agents and environmental pollution.

TIVA can be used in clinical situations where inhalational agents should be avoided (malignant hyperthermia) or where administration of inhalational agents will be difficult (bronchoscopy).

Can you tell me how long it takes for Cp = Ce during a propofol infusion?

About 15 min.

Explain about TCI (target controlled infusion)?

TCI is an infusion system which allows the anaesthetist to select the target blood concentration required for a particular effect. The drug passes from the blood or plasma to the central nervous system (CNS), the effect site, where it exerts its activity. Rapid attainment and maintenance of a constant anaesthetic concentration cannot be achieved accurately using a manually controlled infusion pump, due to the complexity of drug distribution and elimination.

The pharmacokinetic programme of a TCI device, however, continuously calculates the distribution and elimination of the intravenous anaesthetic agent, and successively adjusts the infusion rate to maintain a predicted blood or plasma drug concentration.

The TCI system uses this information to predict the blood or plasma drug concentration associated with the delivery of a given amount of drug. The target drug concentration required to induce and also to maintain anaesthesia is entered into the system by the anaesthetist.

From its pharmacokinetic model, the TCI system determines the initial loading dose needed to achieve the required target concentration and the infusion rate needed to sustain it, and controls the intravenous infusion completely and automatically.

What pharmacokinetic variables are used in calculating the loading dose and maintenance dose in TCI?

The loading dose = the volume of distribution × the desired concentration (i.e. the concentration at steady state).

The maintenance dose is equal to the rate of elimination at steady state (at steady state, rate of elimination = rate of administration):

$$\text{Maintenance dose} = \text{clearance} \times \text{desired plasma concentration.}$$

What do you mean by first-order and zero-order kinetics?

These terms describe the elimination of the drugs from the body.

- *First-order kinetics*: A constant fraction of the drug in the body is eliminated per unit time. The rate of elimination is proportional to the amount of drug in the body. The majority of drugs are eliminated in this way.
- *Zero-order kinetics*: A constant amount of drug is eliminated per unit time. This form of kinetics occurs with several important drugs at high dosage – phenytoin, salicylates, theophylline and thiopentone (at very large doses).

Can you draw me graphs depicting first-order and zero-order kinetics?

The graph shows time on the x-axis and Cp on the y-axis. The graph for first-order kinetic is an exponential curve whereas that of the zero-order kinetics demonstrates a linear relationship.

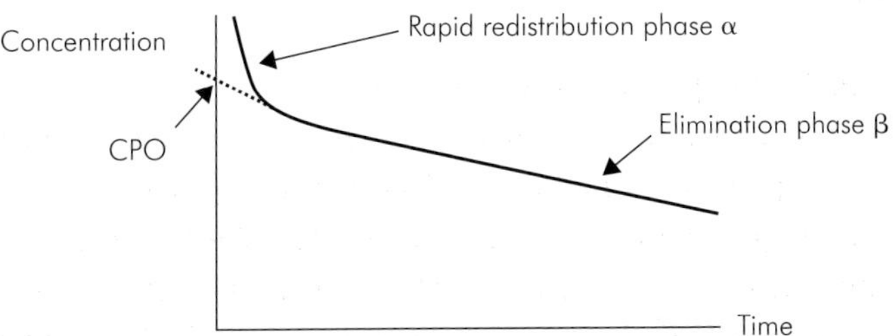

Figure 5.3 *First-order kinetics*

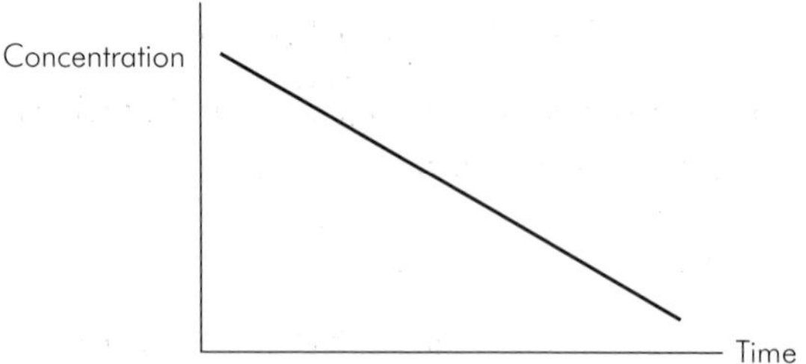

Figure 5.4 *Zero-order kinetics*

What is the Michealis–Menten equation?

The equation is:

$$V = (V_{max} \times Cp)/(K_m + Cp)$$

where V = rate of drug elimination; V_{max} = maximal rate of drug elimination; K_m = affinity constant (affinity of drug for enzyme system); Cp = plasma concentration of drug.

Draw the curve illustrating this equation and explain its significance?

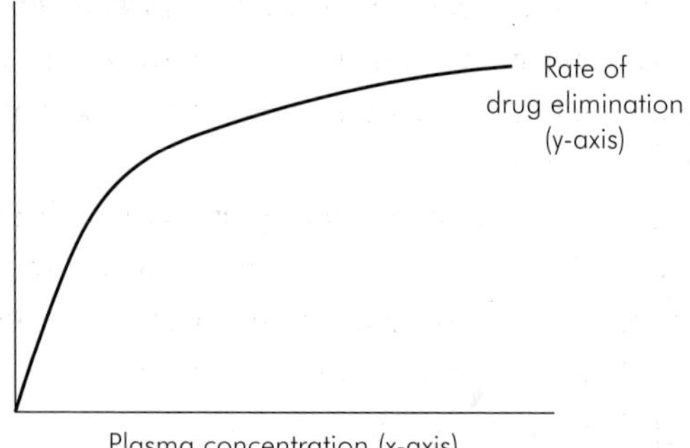

Figure 5.5 *Michealis–Menten equation curve*

In the initial part of the curve, when the Cp is much less than K_m then the above equation can be written as (assuming K_m + Cp = K_m)

$$V = (V_{max} \times Cp)/K_m$$

Or VαCp, that is rate of drug elimination is directly proportional to the drug concentration and it follows first-order kinetics.

However as the drug concentration increases (plateau phase of the curve), the Cp become much greater than K_m and the equation can be written as (on the assumption K_m + Cp = Cp).

$$V = (V_{max} \times Cp)/Cp$$

Or $V \propto V_{max}$ that is rate of drug elimination is constant and equal to maximal rate of drug elimination and it follows zero-order kinetics.

Q3 Hypoglycaemic drugs

What drugs are used to reduce blood sugar in diabetes mellitus?

The hypoglycaemic drugs are broadly classified into two groups:

- Insulin preparations for subcutaneous or intravenous administration,
- Oral hypoglycaemics.

Tell me about insulin.

Insulin is a hormone secreted by the β cells of the Islets of Langerhans in the pancreas. It is a polypeptide containing 51 amino acids arranged in two chains. These are A and B chains linked by disulphide bridges. It has anabolic effects including increased glucose and amino acid uptake, increased glycogenesis, lipogenesis and protein synthesis. It also has anticatabolic effects such as inhibition of lipolysis and protein breakdown. Diabetes mellitus is associated with absolute or relative deficiency of insulin.

What various insulin preparations are you aware of?

Insulin is prepared from porcine or beef pancreas. Now with the advent of recombinant DNA technology human insulin preparations are more commonly used.

Traditionally the preparations are classified based on the duration of action into short, intermediate and long acting.

The duration of action is modified by altering the rate of absorption either by increasing the size of particles or by forming complexes with protamine or zinc.

The onset and duration of action following subcutaneous injection are as follows:

- *Short acting*: Onset 30 min to 1 h; duration up to 8 h.
- *Intermediate acting*: Onset 1–2 h; duration 12–24 h.
- *Long acting*: Onset 2–4 h; duration up to 36 h.

How does insulin act?

Insulin receptors have two α-subunits and two β-subunits linked by disulphide bond. They are membrane spanning glycoproteins. The exact mechanism of action is still unclear. Insulin initially binds to the α-subunit. The insulin–receptor complex enters the cell. After this internalisation the β-subunit exhibits its tyrosine kinase activity and that is how insulin acts.

Can you give a classification for oral hypoglycaemic drugs?

- Sulphonylureas – chlorpropamide, glibenclamide, glimepiride, gliclazide.
- Biguanides – metformin.

- Thiazolidinediones – pioglitazone, rosiglitazone.
- Meglitinide analogues – nateglinide.
- Acarbose.

Can you tell me more about the sulphonylurea group of drugs?

The drugs in this group act by increasing the endogenous insulin secretion from β cells in the pancreas. By blocking the adenosine triphosphate (ATP)-dependent potassium channel they depolarise the membrane of the β cells. As a result calcium influx increases which in turn increases the insulin secretion. Therefore, they require functioning β cells to exert their effect.

These drugs are metabolised in the liver to active metabolites and are eventually excreted in urine. Careful dosage titration is essential as they have a propensity to cause hypoglycaemia.

Sulphonylureas are extensively bound to plasma proteins and hence concurrent administration of other highly protein bound drugs like aspirin can increase the freely available sulphonylurea in the plasma. The group comprises drugs that have a long duration of action such as chlorpropamide (1–3 days) as well as those with a shorter duration of action such as tolbutamide (5 h).

How does the action of biguanides differ from sulphonylureas?

Unlike sulphonylureas biguanides have no effect on insulin secretion. They act peripherally by increasing the sensitivity of the tissues to insulin.

What is the main concern in using biguanides?

They carry a risk of lactic acidosis. This may possibly due to inhibition of oxidative phosphorylation at the cellular level.

Clinical 5

Key topics: APLS, stridor, malignant hyperthermia (MH)

Q1 An 8-year-old girl has been brought into the resuscitation room following a road traffic accident. She has already been intubated and ventilated. You are called to see her

How will you proceed with this case?

My approach will be airway, breathing and circulation:

- *Airway*: As she is already intubated, confirm the placement of the endotracheal tube, observe chest movements and monitor end tidal carbon dioxide ($ETCO_2$) trace.

- *Breathing*: Assess adequacy of ventilation, respiratory rate, listen for breath sounds and check whether they are equal both the sides, chest expansion, $ETCO_2$. Look for effects of inadequate ventilation – heart rate, skin colour, SpO_2.
- *Circulation*: Check heart rate, blood pressure (BP), peripheral circulation and capillary filling.

Look at results of primary and secondary surveys. Consider need for scans, cervical spine films and/or neurosurgical referral if appropriate.

How can you calculate the approximate size and length of the endotracheal tube in paediatrics?

- *Size*: (Age/4) + 4.
- *Length*: (Age/2) + 12 for oral tubes, (Age/2 + 14) for nasal tubes.

Tell me about assessment of her circulation.

Cardiovascular status can be assessed by considering heart rate and rhythm, pulse volume, capillary refill, BP, temperature, urine output.

How will you look for capillary refill? What is the significance of this testing?

Capillary refill is a guide to skin perfusion. Poor skin perfusion can be a useful early sign of shock. Capillary refill is tested on the skin of the sternum or a digit held at the level of the heart. Normal refill time is less than 2 s after blanching pressure for 5 s. In early shock, even when the circulation is hyperdynamic due to vasodilatation in which the peripheries are warm, the capillary refill may still be delayed indicating poor peripheral perfusion.

What are the shortcomings of BP measurement as a sign of adequate circulation?

Measurement and interpretation of BP is difficult in small children. The child cardiovascular system can compensate well for blood loss. Hypotension is a late and often sudden sign of decompensation. Presence of tachycardia may be a cardinal sign.

How can you calculate blood volume?

Circulating blood volume in children is about 80 ml/kg.

Tell me about fluid resuscitation in this child.

Fluids are used in resuscitation where perfusion is compromised. Assessment of perfusion is challenging and relies on assessment of organ function – urine output, mentation, peripheral perfusion. If the child is in shock:

Two boluses of 20 ml/kg make 40 ml/kg which is roughly half of the circulating blood volume. If the shock is persistent after first two boluses due consideration should be given to blood transfusion. Further management depends on factors such as the amount of previous blood loss, degree of shock and ongoing blood loss.

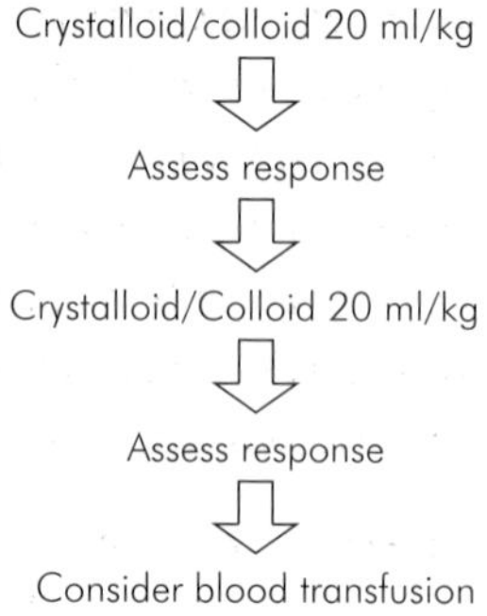

Crystalloid/colloid 20 ml/kg
⇩
Assess response
⇩
Crystalloid/Colloid 20 ml/kg
⇩
Assess response
⇩
Consider blood transfusion

Q2 Critical incident: airway obstruction

Alright! This child is very stable now after resuscitation and you have decided to extubate. Immediately following the extubation she develops noisy breathing and starts desaturating. How will you manage?

Noisy breathing is usually due to airway obstruction. Call for senior help and in the mean time try and resolve the situation. Diagnosis and management of the condition should go hand with hand. First assess the adequacy of ventilation to decide if the tube should be resited.

Ok, but what could be the possible causes?

The noisy breathing, stridor, can be inspiratory or expiratory.

Inspiratory stridor is usually due to upper airway obstruction which can either be at the level of oropharynx or at larynx.

Table 5.1 *Causes of upper airway obstruction in the postoperative period*

	Oropharyngeal obstruction	Laryngeal obstruction
Common	Decrease muscle tone	Laryngospasm
	Secretions	Secretions
	Sleep apnoea	
Rare	Foreign body	Oedema
	Oedema	Bilateral recurrent laryngeal nerve palsy
	Wound haematoma	Tracheal collapse
	Neuromuscular disease	

Expiratory obstruction can be due to:

- Inhaled foreign body.
- Inhalational injury.
- Aspiration.
- Secretions.
- Incidental wheeze, asthma, etc.

How will you manage stridor following upper airway obstruction?

Administer 100% oxygen. Closing the pressure limiting valve can provide continuous positive airway pressure (CPAP) and will be beneficial if it is laryngospasm. Head tilt and jaw thrust can open the airway. Clearing the secretions and turning the patient to the recovery position can be helpful. Simple airway adjuncts like oropharyngeal airway (if the jaw is relaxed) or nasopharyngeal airway (if the jaw is closed tight) may be of use in relieving the obstruction.

With all these manoeuvre if the obstruction is not relieved what else will you do?

Propofol is useful to break the spasm and take control over airway. Suxamethonium in smaller dose (0.1–0.2 mg/kg intravenously) has been advocated. Alternatively normal dose of 1–2 mg/kg intravenously has been used to facilitate full relaxation followed by orotracheal intubation.

Alternatively if there is a definitive cause for airway obstruction, like a wound haematoma, it needs to be drained. If none of these interventions help and mask ventilation with 100% oxygen is impossible then a surgical airway will be required.

Q3 Malignant hyperthermia

Tell me what you know about malignant hyperthermia (MH)?

MH is an acute pharmacogenetic disorder, with autosomal-dominant inheritance. Both genetic predisposition and one or more triggering agents are necessary to evoke MH.

Can you name some triggering agents?

Triggering agents include all volatile anaesthetics (halothane, enflurane, isoflurane, sevoflurane, desflurane) and depolarising muscle relaxants (suxamethonium).

What is the incidence of MH?

The prevalence of the genetic MH predisposition is between 1:5000 and 1:10,000; the incidence of reported MH reactions varies from 1 in 40,000 to 1 in 100,000 anaesthetics.

Can you describe the pathogenesis of MH?

Volatile anaesthetics and/or suxamethonium cause a raise in the myoplasmic calcium concentration. The raise in calcium concentration leads to an activation of actin and myosin filaments and explains the rigidity and the masseter spasm – early signs of MH. The raised calcium concentration further leads to a stimulation of the energy consuming processes in the skeletal muscle, leading to a metabolic acidosis. There is uncontrolled oxidative phosphorylation. The hypermetabolism seen in MH leads to several clinical signs like hypertonia, arrhythmia, tachycardia and hyperthermia. Acidosis results from excessive production of carbon dioxide and lactic acid. Rhabdomyolysis occurs as a result of excessive contractile activity. Laboratory findings include hyperkalaemia, raised creatine kinase and myoglobinuria.

Some MH families showed a defect on chromosome 19, on the ryanodine receptor gene. Ryanodine, an alkaloid, binds selectively to the ryanodine receptor, a calcium channel in the sarcoplasmic reticulum. Other families with MH predisposition showed no ryanodine receptor defect. Due to this heterogenecity it is difficult to perform an MH test, based on genetics.

What are the clinical presentations of MH?

MH has a wide spectrum of presentation:

- *Muscle rigidity*: This can be isolated masseter spasm or generalised rigidity.
- *Classical MH crisis*: Due to hypermetabolism there is an unexplained increase in $ETCO_2$ and tachycardia; later a rise in body temperature that can exceed a rate of more than 1°C/10 min. Eventually because of extensive cellular damage hyperkalaemia, increased plasma creatine kinase and myoglobinuria ensues. Acidosis can be severe. Arrhythmias and disseminated intravascular coagulation are other features.
- Other miscellaneous presentations include postoperative acute renal failure due to myoglobinuria, unexpected cardiac arrest or even death.

How will you manage a case of MH crisis?

Early recognition and immediate intervention are mandatory for a successful outcome.

- Stop triggering agent, remove vaporiser.
- Hyperventilation with 100% oxygen.
- Deepen anaesthesia with intravenous drugs; muscle relaxation with a non-depolarising relaxant.
- Stop surgery as soon as possible.
- Monitor temperature; active cooling measures.
- Dantrolene 3 mg/kg intravenously repeated up to a dose of 10 mg/kg until tachycardia and rise in $ETCO_2$ subsides.
- Acidosis and hyperkalaemia need prompt addressing with sodium bicarbonate and dextrose insulin infusion respectively.
- Send blood for arterial blood gas analysis, urea and electrolytes.
- Antiarrhythmic therapy for arrhythmias.
- Additional monitoring: arterial catheter, central venous catheter, urinary catheter.
- Maintain hydration and ensure good diuresis with fluids and mannitol. Alkalinising the urine helps in myoglobinuria.
- Check for serum creatine kinase, clotting abnormalities.

- Postoperative intensive care/high dependency unit.
- Inform patient, relatives and general practitioner, test patient and relatives for MH susceptibility in an MH diagnostic centre (in vitro contracture test), if positive: MH susceptibility identity card.

How will you anaesthetise a young adult with a strong family history of MH now requiring urgent surgery for fractured shaft of femur?

Firstly, the general principles of preoperative visit which will include eliciting detailed history, examination and investigation. The patient should be stabilised as he might have lost considerable amount of blood and may have sustained other injuries. Liaise with the surgeon to establish the urgency of the procedure.

Assuming he has isolated fracture shaft of femur and has been tested susceptible for MH, what will be your choice of anaesthesia?

If there is no contraindication regional anaesthesia is an ideal option to avoid the problems associated with multiple pharmacological agents used in providing general anaesthesia. This can either be spinal, epidural or a combined spinal epidural depending on the tentative duration of the procedure.

If you have to provide general anaesthesia what precautions will you take?

Triggering drugs should be avoided. If the department has an MH-safe vapour free machine it should be used. Otherwise a machine can be prepared by removal of vaporisers and flushing through the machine and ventilator with 100% oxygen at maximal flow for about 30 min. A fresh breathing circuit must be used. Standard monitoring including electrocardiogram (ECG), pulse oximetry, capnography and temperature measurement is necessary. Ensure dantrolene is readily available. If the patient has an aspiration risk, perform a modified rapid sequence induction with rocuronium as relaxant. Anaesthesia can be maintained with intravenous agents.

Can you list some drugs used in anaesthetic practice that are safe in MH patients?

All intravenous anaesthetics including ketamine and benzodiazepines are safe. All analgesics and non-depolarising muscle relaxants are safe. Nitrous oxide has been safely used. Other safe drugs include local anaesthetics, neostigmine, atropine and glycopyrrolate.

What are the tests available for confirming the diagnosis of MH?

The mainstay of diagnosis is in vitro contracture testing. Muscle biopsy is taken from vastus muscle and exposed to halothane and caffeine. The tension generated in the muscle is higher in patients susceptible to develop MH. The test result can be MH susceptible, MH equivocal or MH negative depending on whether the test is positive with both halothane and caffeine, either of them or neither of them respectively.

What other conditions can simulate MH?

- Light plane of anaesthesia and inadequate analgesia.
- Anaphylaxis.
- Sepsis.
- Thyroid storm.
- Phaeochromocytoma.
- Neuroleptic malignant syndrome and other muscle diseases.

Physics, clinical measurement and safety 5

Key topics: cylinders, oxygen storage, electrical symbols, defibrillator and scavenging

Q1 Cylinders

How do you identify an oxygen cylinder?

It is colour coded, body is black in colour and shoulder is white.

			Colour coding	
Substance	Gas/Vapour	Symbol	Cylinder	Shoulder
Oxygen	Gas	O_2	Black	White
Air	Gas	AIR	Black	White/black
Nitrous oxide	Vapour	N_2O	Blue	Blue
Entonox	Gas and vapour	N_2O/O_2	Blue	White/blue
Carbon dioxide	Vapour	CO_2	Grey	Grey
Helium	Gas	He	Brown	Brown

Figure 5.6 *Colour coding of gas cylinders (for UK and ISO)*

What other information is written on the gas cylinders?

The name and symbol of the gas contained is stencilled both on the shoulder and on the valve block. Each cylinder has a unique serial number. The shape and colour of the plastic test disc indicates the quarter and the year in which the cylinder was last tested. Cylinder size code, tare weight of the cylinder, hydraulic test pressure of the cylinder, owner and manufacturer of the gas is also written on the cylinder. The label on the cylinder also includes hazard warnings and safety instructions.

What is the size of the oxygen cylinder that is commonly used on the anaesthetic machines?
Size E.

What is the pressure in the oxygen cylinder when it is full?
The pressure within a full 'E' size cylinder is 137 bar (1980 psi). It is capable of supplying 670 l of oxygen at room temperature.

What is the pressure in the oxygen cylinder, when it is half empty? Why? How does it differ from a nitrous oxide cylinder?
It is half the original pressure, 68.5 bar. When a non-liquefied compressed gas such as oxygen is discharged the pressure in the cylinder declines steadily (Boyle's law). With gases stored partially in the liquid form (nitrous oxide), the pressure gauge shows a constant pressure (at constant temperature) until all the liquid has evaporated, after this there is a steady decline in pressure as the gas is used up. The gauge pressure cannot be used to estimate contents, but the weight will decline steadily during use.

Content	Gas/Vapour	Cylinder pressure kPa (psi)	BP at 1 atm (°C)	Critical Temperature (°C)
Oxygen	Gas	13,700 (1980)	−183	−118
Air	Gas	13,700 (1980)		
Nitrous oxide	Vapour	4400 (640)	−89	36.5
Carbon dioxide	Vapour	5000 (723)	−78.5	31
Entonox	Mixture	13,700 (1980)	Gas separation at −6 °C	
Helium	Gas	13,700 (1980)	−269	−268

Figure 5.7 *Gases and vapours supplied in cylinders*

What precautions do you take when attaching a cylinder to the anaesthetic machine?
First confirm identity of the cylinder and inspect the cylinder for any damage.

The plastic dust cover from valve block should be removed. The valve should be slightly opened and closed (cracked) to clear the dust particles, oil and grease from the exit port. A Bodok seal must be placed between the exit port of cylinder and the inlet port of yoke of the anaesthetic machine. The cylinder valve should be opened slowly initially and once the pressure gauge has stabilised it can be opened fully. Check that the gauge pressure is appropriate and there are no leaks.

What is a pin index system and why it is used?

It is a safety system used to prevent the interchangeability of the cylinders. A specific pin configuration exists on the inlet part (yoke) of the anaesthetic machine. There are holes on the valve block of the cylinder which should match the pins on the yoke. Unless this matches, a cylinder cannot be fitted into the anaesthetic machine.

What are these cylinders made of?

Cylinders are made of molybdenum steel. Small size cylinders are also made of aluminium alloy with a fibre glass covering.

How are these cylinders tested?

Hydraulic pressure testing is carried out every 5 years using water under high pressure. Each cylinder is subjected to a pressure considerably greater than that would be required in clinical use. Test pressure is stencilled on the valve block of the cylinder.

One out of every 100 cylinders manufactured is tensile tested. Strips are cut from the body and stretched to assess the yield point.

Cylinders can be inspected endoscopically for any cracks and defects on their inner surfaces. Flattening, bend and impact tests are carried out on at least one out of 100 cylinders.

How else is oxygen stored?

Oxygen is also stored in the liquid form in vacuum-insulated evaporators (VIE). This consists of an inner stainless steel tank and an outer steel jacket. The temperature inside is −160 to −180°C (lower than the critical temperature of oxygen which is −118°C). There is a main outlet at the top of the VIE, from which the oxygen is supplied to the pipelines. A pressure regulator allows the pressure to be reduced to four bar before entering the pipelines. A safety valve opens at 17 bar if the pressure builds up when oxygen is not used. When there is increased demand, oxygen is also withdrawn from a separate outlet at the bottom. This liquid oxygen is evaporated by passing through the super heater.

Oxygen supplied in gaseous form through a dedicated copper pipeline network leading to Schraeder wall outlets which accept non-interchangeable Schraeder probes that are attached to named and colour coded gas hoses.

How can you extract oxygen from air?

Oxygen concentrators extract oxygen from air. An air compressor drives filtered air through zeolite columns (hydrated aluminium silicate which acts as a molecular sieve) which retains nitrogen. The maximum oxygen concentration achieved is 95%.

Concentrators require only electricity and minimal servicing, are reliable and provide a continuous supply of oxygen.

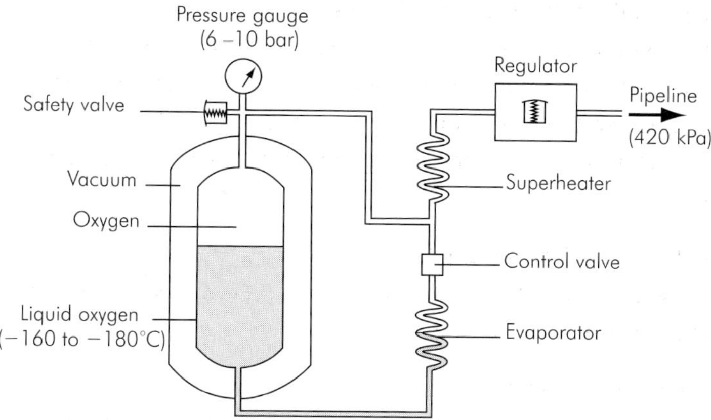

Figure 5.8 *Vacuum insulated evaporator*

Q2 Electrical symbols and defibrillator

Can you name the following electrical symbols?

- *Resistor*: used in an electrical circuit to reduce the voltage or current.
- *Capacitor*: a component which stores electric charge.
- *Inductor*: made by forming a conductor into coils, which are often wound round a core of ferrous material. It produces a concentrated magnetic field.
- *Diode*: a semiconductor which only enables current to flow through it in one direction. It is often used to convert alternating current (AC) to direct current (DC) in order to provide DC power supply.
- *Transformer*: used to transform the AC voltage, either to step up or step down the AC voltages in the circuit. It consists of two coils, a primary, for the input and a secondary, for the output, wound on a common iron core. The change in voltage depends on the number of turns in the primary and secondary winding.
- *Transistor*: a semiconductor device used to amplify small current signals.

What is capacitance?

Capacitance describes the property of a device enabling it to store electrical charge. A capacitor consists of two conducting plates separated by a thin layer of insulating material.

Can you give an example of interference caused by capacitance?

Interference in the electrocardiogram (ECG) trace produced from the AC passing through the operating theatre light.

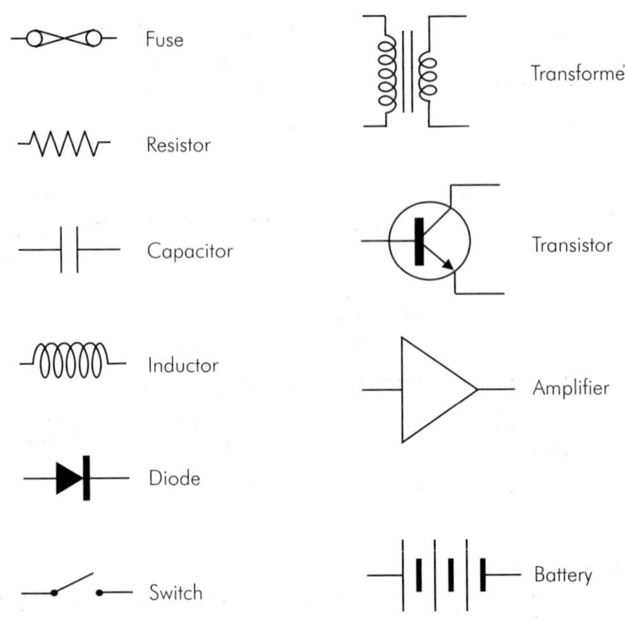

Figure 5.9 *Circuit symbols*

A capacitor will allow the AC to pass in the gap between the two plates. In an operating theatre, the theatre lamp acts as one plate of the capacitor and the patient as the other plate. A small amount of 50 Hz – AC current passes from the lamp to the patient resulting in interference on the ECG trace.

What is a defibrillator?

It is a piece of electrical equipment in which electric charge is stored and released in a controlled fashion.

How does it work?

It has a *power* source from the mains or from a battery. A *rectifier* (diode) is used to convert alternate current into DC.

Electric charge is stored in a *capacitor*, which consists of two plates separated by an insulator. When the defibrillator is activated, it releases the stored charge.

An *inductor* is included in the output circuit which lengthens the duration of current pulse. This inductor in the discharge path opposes sudden change in current flow, slows down the rapid discharge from the capacitor and hence controls the duration of the shock. It also absorbs some of the electrical charge, hence the delivered energy is less than that of stored energy. Energy indicated on the defibrillator is the actual delivered energy, not the stored energy. Maximum energy delivered in the monophasic defibrillator is normally 360 J.

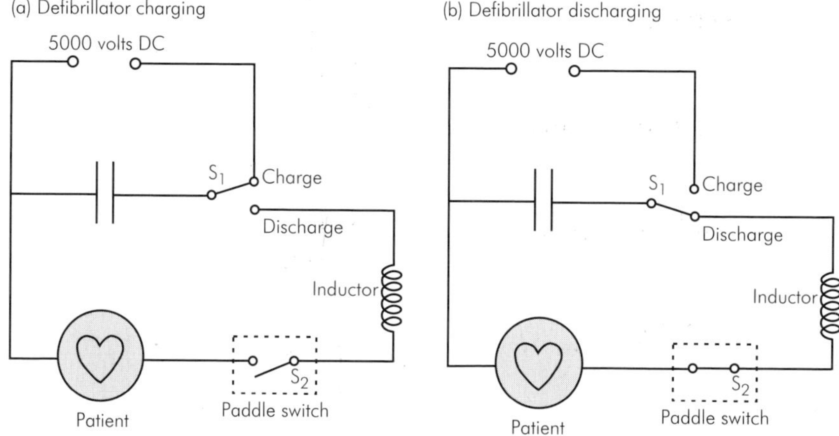

Figure 5.10 *Defibrillator circuit (a) charging (b) discharging, through patient*

How do you calculate the stored energy?

Stored energy, E = ½QV, where Q is the charge in millicoulombs and V is the potential (volts).

How does biphasic differ from monophasic defibrillator?

Monophasic defibrillator produces single pulse of current which travels in one direction through the chest. Biphasic defibrillator produces two consecutive pulses, in which the current first travels in one direction and then in the other. In the biphasic type, defibrillation threshold is lower than in a monophasic defibrillator and hence it is more efficient.

Q3 Scavenging

What are the principle sources of pollution in the operating theatre?

Expired gases from the spill valve of the breathing system, leaks from equipment, gases exhaled from the patient while transfer to recovery and spillage from filling of vaporisers can pollute the operating theatre environment.

What is the maximum permitted level of nitrous oxide and other anaesthetic vapours as a pollutant?

It is 100 ppm for nitrous oxide. The maximum acceptable levels are 10 ppm for halothane and 50 ppm for enflurane and isoflurane.

How can we prevent theatre pollution?

- Use of circle systems reduces the potential for atmospheric pollution.
- Air conditioning. Rapid air change in theatre reduces pollution substantially, but some systems recycle air.

- Vaporisers should be filled with optimum care to avoid any spillage.
- Appropriate use of scavenging system will prevent theatre pollution.
- Using total intravenous anaesthesia (TIVA).
- Practicing regional anaesthesia.

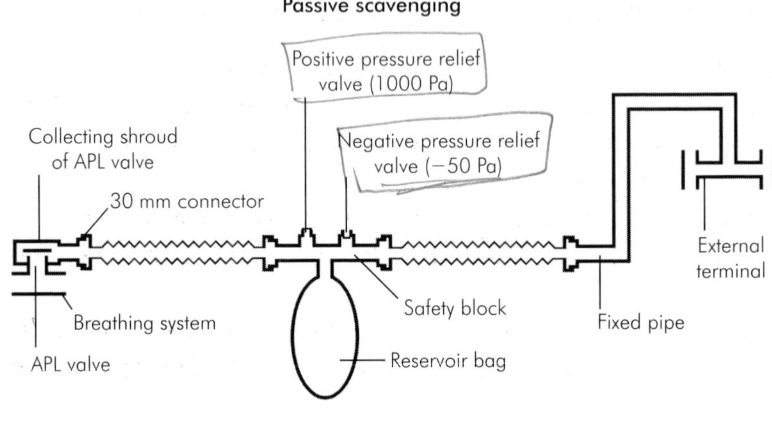

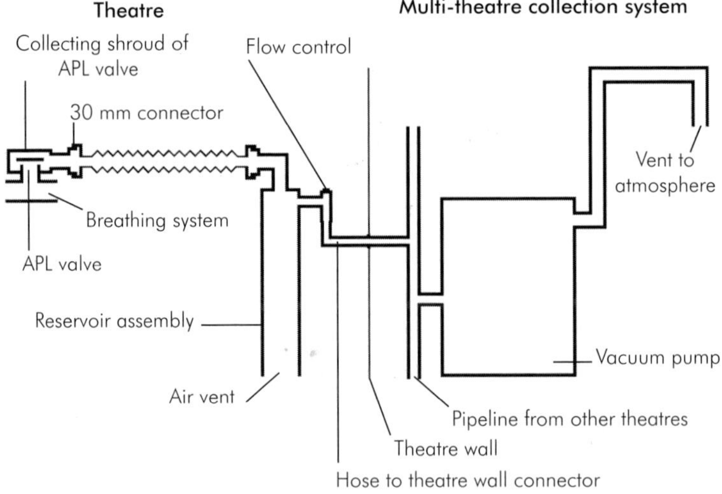

Figure 5.11 *Scavenging systems*

Can you classify scavenging systems and describe the features of each of them?

Active systems: These generate a negative pressure which propels gases to the outside atmosphere. These may be powered by a vacuum pump or may use a venturi system to create subatmospheric pressure. The components of active system include a collecting system, a receiving system and a disposal system.

The collecting and transfer system consists of tubing connected to the adjustable pressure limiting valve using a 30 mm connector. The receiving system consists of an open ended reservoir which houses a visual flow indicator. The active disposal system consists of a fan or a pump used to generate a vacuum. The system should operate with a pressure of −0.5 and +5 cmH_2O. The system should be capable of accommodating 75 l/min continuous flow with a peak of 130 l/min.

What problems may be expected with active systems system?

Excessive negative pressure may lead to collapse of the reservoir bag of the breathing system and may lead to rebreathing. Excessive positive pressure from the system may lead to barotrauma.

Semi-active systems: Waste gases conducted to the extraction side of the air-conditioning system, which generates a small negative pressure within the scavenging tubing.

Passive systems: The patient's expiratory effort or the pressure from the ventilator propels the waste gas down an additional length of tubing to the outside atmosphere.

Pressure within the system may be altered by the wind conditions at the external terminal (may generate a negative pressure but also a high positive pressure is possible).

Physiology 6

Key topics: cardiac physiology, altitude, starvation

Q1 Cardiac cycle and cardiac pump

Can you draw a cardiac cycle showing the left ventricular pressure over time? Please superimpose the aortic pressure and atrial pressure waveforms in your diagram.

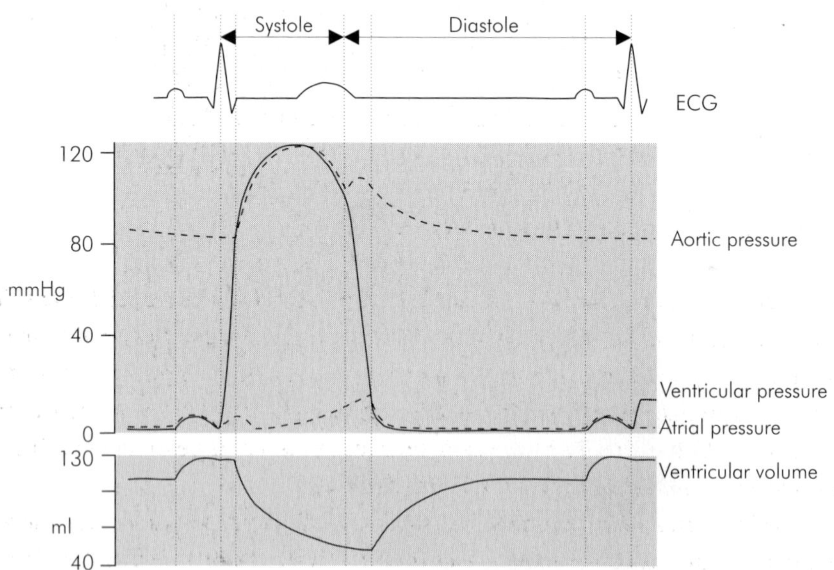

Figure 6.1 *Cardiac cycle showing ventricular volume, ventricular pressure, aortic pressure and atrial pressure*

What are the various stages during systole and diastole?

Systole can further be divided into two stages:

1 Isovolumetric contraction.

2 Ejection.

Diastole is divided into four stages:

1 Isovolumetric relaxation.

2 Rapid ventricular filling.

3 Diastasis (slow ventricular filling).

4 Atrial contraction.

Draw me a pressure-volume loop for the ventricle.

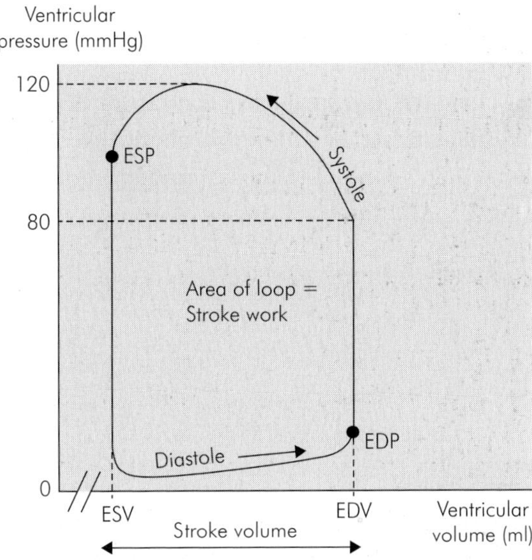

Figure 6.2 *Pressure–volume loop for the ventricle*

At the end-diastolic point (EDP) the atrio-ventricular valves (mitral and tricuspid) close (first heart sound). The semilunar valves (aortic and pulmonary) have not yet opened and isovolumetric contraction occurs increasing the pressure within the ventricle. The ejection phase commences with the opening of the semilunar valves and lasts until the closure of the semilunar valves (second heart sound). This is marked as the end-systolic point (ESP) in the loop.

Diastole begins with the isovolumetric relaxation phase where both atrio-ventricular valves and semilunar valves remain closed. There is a sharp drop in the pressure within the ventricles. The flatter portion in the base of the loop represents the rest of the diastole – rapid ventricular filling after the opening of atrio-ventricular valves, diastasis and atrial contraction. Diastole ends in the EDP with the closure of atrio-ventricular valves and the cycle completes.

What are the various components of the central venous pressure (CVP) waveform and what do they reflect?

The CVP waveform reflects the pressure changes in the right atrium and has three positive deflections (a, c and v) and two negative deflections (x and y).

They represent:

a: **a**trial contraction

c: isovolumetric contraction (corresponds to **c**arotid pulse)

v: atrial filling with **v**enous blood

x: pulmonary valve opens, fall in right ventricular pressure, atrium rela**x**es

y: emp**ty**ing of atrial blood into ventricle.

What is the Frank–Starling law?

The Frank–Starling law states that the force of contraction of cardiac muscle is proportional to its initial length. In the heart, within physiological limits, an increase in end-diastolic volume (EDV) produces a more forceful contraction and an increase in stroke volume (SV).

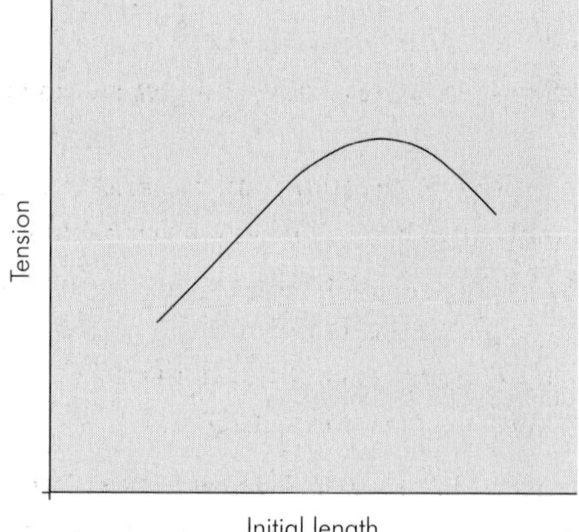

Figure 6.3 *Frank curve for isolated muscle fibre*

Why does the curve descend beyond a limit? What are the various factors that can move the position of Frank–Starling curve?

The normal length of sarcomere is about 2.2 μm and during optimal filling pressure they are compliant and follow the Frank–Starling relationship – an increase in SV with increase in filling pressure. Even if the filling pressure progressively increases the sarcomere length cannot increase beyond 2.6 μm and hence the curve starts descending.

Cardiac failure, beta-blockers, hypoxia and acidosis causes a right and downward shift. Sympathetic stimulation and ionotropes can shift the curve upwards and to the left improving contractility.

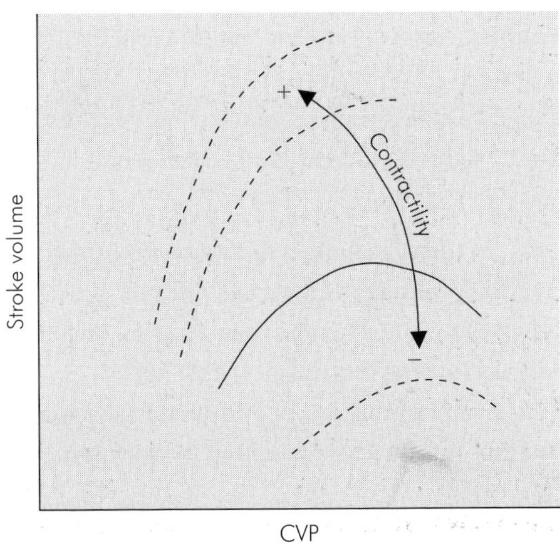

Figure 6.4 *Ventricular function curve*

Q2 High altitude

What physiological changes take place if a person climbs up to an altitude of 5500 m?

At high altitude there is a significant drop in the barometric pressure (at 5500 m the barometric pressure is about half the value at sea level), but the fraction of oxygen in the atmospheric air remains the same ($F_IO_2 = 0.21$). Thus there is a reduction in the partial pressure of inspired oxygen (P_IO_2).

A series of physiological changes take place, both on a short term and long-term basis to counter this fall in the inspired oxygen tension.

Tell me in detail about the changes pertaining to the respiratory system.

Secondary to the fall in P_IO_2 there is a fall in alveolar oxygen tension as well resulting arterial hypoxemia [$P_AO_2 = P_IO_2 - P_ACO_2/RQ$].

Hypoxia stimulates the peripheral chemoreceptors (location: aortic and carotid bodies) leading to hyperventilation. Alveolar ventilation increases by 4–5 times. This effectively washes out the carbon dioxide causing a considerable drop in P_ACO_2. Again, this has an influence in the alveolar gas equation which leads to a rise in P_AO_2 which will be compatible with survival. This is an immediate response. Later there is a more gradual increase in hyperventilation due to renal elimination of bicarbonate, bicarbonate shift out of cerebrospinal fluid (CSF) and desensitisation of central chemoreceptors.

There is increased pulmonary arterial pressure due to hypoxic pulmonary vasoconstriction. This higher pulmonary arterial pressure and lower alveolar pressure together contribute to more even distribution of perfusion through the lung. There is better ventilation–perfusion matching. Diffusion capacity of lungs increases (normal is 21 ml/mmHg/min) due to increased capillary blood volume and an increase in lung volume.

On acclimatisation 2,3 Diphosphoglycerate (2, 3-DPG) increases, oxygen dissociation curve shifts to the right, P_{50} increases and there is better oxygen delivery to the tissues.

What are the various circulatory changes due to acclimatisation?

Hyperplasia of erythroid cells and increased red cell production lead to polycythemia. Haemoglobin levels reach more than 20 g/100 ml helping to enhance the oxygen content of blood to more than 22 ml O_2/100 ml.

Hypoxia results in local vasodilatation. Peripheral tissues show an increase in capillary density. Cardiac output and circulating blood volume increase.

What do you mean by high altitude pulmonary oedema. When does it occur?

High altitude pulmonary oedema can develop within 6 h of rapid ascent to high altitude. The risk factors include elderly people, existing chronic obstructive airway disease (COAD) and those with SaO_2 less than 90%.

The various proposed mechanisms include:

- Increased hydrostatic pressure.
- Increased permeability due to capillary endothelial damage as result of increased resistance, increased viscosity, and increased cardiac output.
- Release of vasoactive mediators secondary to hypoxia.
- Increased free radicals in skeletal muscles, and visceral organs.

What is acute mountain sickness?

Rapid ascent to an altitude above 2500 m can result in acute mountain sickness. The symptoms include exertional dyspnoea, headache, nausea, insomnia, and muscle fatigue. Cheyne–Stokes breathing and sleep apnoea occurs at altitude above 4000 m. Acute mountain sickness is thought to be due to acute hypoxia and alkalosis. In severe cases pulmonary or cerebral oedemas ensue.

Q3 Starvation

What do you mean by starvation? Can you tell me what happens if someone starves for several days?

Starvation is complete absence of dietary intake.

Various metabolic changes take place in order to meet the glucose requirements. Later, most of the organs in the body adapt to utilise alternate sources of fuel.

What is the average body reserve of fuels during total starvation?

- *Carbohydrate*: About 500 g of reserve is available in the form of glycogen in liver and muscle. Glycogenolysis is sufficient to meet the glucose requirements for the first 24 h following starvation thereby avoiding protein or fat breakdown.
- *Protein*: This provides amino acids that are utilised in gluconeogenesis. About 5 kg of protein is stored in the muscle which can last for up to 2 weeks.
- *Fat*: In long-term starvation this forms the most important source for fuel and it is stored in the form of adipose tissues. In an average there is about 10–15 kg fat available for breakdown that will provide energy substrate for 4 weeks.

Describe in detail the metabolic changes that follow starvation in a chronological sequence.

Initially there is an increase in glycogenolysis, which provides glucose. The brain is mainly dependent on glucose as an energy substrate and hence meeting its glucose requirement gets first priority. Once the glycogen store is depleted and glucose levels start falling fatty acids are mobilised. Liver and muscle start using fatty acids as energy source, sparing glucose for the brain.

With total depletion of glycogen reserve, amino acids (derived from the breakdown of muscle protein) and glycerol (derived from fat) are used in the process of gluconeogenesis to produce glucose. This takes place in the liver.

Most tissues, including the brain, ultimately adapt to use ketone bodies as a fuel source. Acetyl-CoA produced during fatty acid metabolism accumulates, resulting in ketosis.

What you mean by the protein sparing effect of glucose?

During starvation, protein catabolism can be counteracted by providing a small amount of glucose. Glucose stimulates the release of insulin secretion which inhibits the breakdown of protein in muscle.

In starvation, although there is an initial rapid protein catabolism, later as the ketone bodies are used as energy source, the rate of protein catabolism decreases.

Pharmacology 6

Key topics: benzodiazepines, blood–brain barrier, pK and ionisation, anticholinesterases

Q1 Benzodiazepines

Which benzodiazepines do you use commonly?

Diazepam, midazolam, temazepam, lorazepam.

What is the mode of action of benzodiazepines?

Benzodiazepines enhance GABA mediated inhibitory transmission at $GABA_A$ receptors. These receptors are widespread in the cortex and the limbic system of the central nervous system (CNS). Benzodiazepines act by increasing the affinity of GABA for the receptor. By facilitating the effects of GABA (the main inhibitory neurotransmitter in CNS) there is an increase in the frequency of chloride channel opening. The presence of the anion chloride causes hyperpolarisation of the cells and the transmission of impulses is inhibited.

Tell me more about the GABA receptors.

GABA receptors are widely scattered in the CNS wherever the inhibitory neurotransmitter GABA acts. At least two distinct group of receptors are identified, $GABA_A$ and $GABA_B$.

$GABA_A$ receptors are integral membrane proteins. They have a pentameric structure with α-, β- and γ-subunits. GABA acts on the α- and β- subunits to open the chloride channels in the $GABA_A$ receptors resulting in neuronal hyperpolarisation and inhibition. Benzodiazepines appear to act on α and γ subunits. Various anaesthetic drugs are thought to exert their effect by acting on $GABA_A$ receptors. Etomidate binds with the β subunit.

$GABA_A$ receptors are predominantly found in the cortex and the limbic system though they can also be identified in brain stem and in spinal cord.

The second distinct group is the $GABA_B$ receptor. They are located primarily in the brain stem and spinal cord though can also be identified elsewhere in CNS. This type of receptor is coupled to G proteins (G_i) and adenylate cyclase. Receptor activation decrease cyclic adenosine mono phosphate (cAMP) and subsequent reduction in the release of neuropeptides and other excitatory neurotransmitters. Baclofen is a specific analogue of GABA at $GABA_B$ receptors. It is used to relieve spasm in neurological disorders.

What is the significance of the structure of midazolam?

The ring structure of midazolam changes with the surrounding pH. In an ampoule at an acidic pH of 4, midazolam is ionised in aqueous solution and is water soluble. The ring is open.

The pH of plasma alters the structure of midazolam. At pH 7.4 the ring closes increasing its lipid solubility.

Can you compare and contrast midazolam with diazepam?

Table 6.1 *Midazolam and diazepam*

Property	Diazepam	Midazolam
Structure	1,4 benzodiazepine	Imidazobenzodiazepine.
Solubility	Insoluble in water	Soluble in water
Presentation	Lipid emulsion	Aqueous preparation
Pain on injection	Yes	No
Pharmacokinetics		
pH	6.4–6.9	3 to 4
Protein binding (%)	96–98	94
Elimination half-life (hours)	24–48	1–3
Metabolism		
Active metabolites	Yes	No
	N-demethylation to form desmethyl diazepam, then hydroxylated to oxazepam	Hydroxylated to hydroxymidazolam
Pharmacodynamics		
Onset of action	Slow	Fast
Anterograde amnesia	++	++++
Duration	Longer	Shorter
Feto/maternal ratio	High	Low

Can you list some uses of benzodiazepines?

- Anxiolysis.
- Hypnotic – sleep disorders.
- Antiepileptic.
- Delirium tremens.
- Centrally acting muscle relaxant in spastic conditions.
- Premedication.
- Co-induction of anaesthesia.
- Sedation for procedures (endoscopy).
- Sedation in intensive care unit.

What are the unwanted effects associated with the use of benzodiazepines?

- Pain on injection with diazepam.
- Impaired psychomotor performance.
- Hangover effects.
- Can cause serious ventilatory depression.
- Risk of tolerance, drug dependence and substance abuse.

- Rapid eye movement (REM) sleep is considerably reduced. On cessation of treatment with benzodiazepines there is a rebound phenomenon with increased duration spent in REM sleep and hence unpleasant dreams and nightmares.

How can you antagonise the action of benzodiazepines?
Intravenous administration of the competitive antagonist flumazenil can be used to reverse the action of benzodiazepines. As it has a short duration of action with an elimination half-life of about 50 min, patients need to be carefully monitored to observe the re-emergence of benzodiazepine effects. Flumazenil can also provoke withdrawal effects in patients receiving benzodiazepines on long-term basis.

Can you tell me more about flumazenil?
It is an imidazobenzodiazepine like midazolam. It is a benzodiazepine receptor antagonist with a high-hepatic extraction ratio and a short duration of action. About 40–50% of the drug is protein bound. It is initially given in a dose of 0.2 mg with further increments until recovery is complete.

It can precipitate convulsions in epileptic patients which can be due to its inverse agonist effects at $GABA_A$ receptors.

What do you mean by inverse agonist?
Inverse agonists are drugs with receptor affinity but negative intrinsic activity.

Q2 Drugs and the blood–brain barrier

What is the 'blood–brain barrier'?
The blood–brain barrier is a dynamic interface between the blood and brain that restricts free transfer of certain chemicals between blood and brain. It has a structural component and a metabolic component.

What is its structure?
The 'structural barrier' is made of tight junctions by the overlapping endothelial cells in the cerebral capillaries. These capillaries are further surrounded by a basement membrane which is closely adherent to the neuroglial cells – astrocytes. These structures, endothelium, basement membrane and astrocytes collectively form a structural barrier. It prevents free passage of some drugs by simple diffusion or filtration from blood into the CNS.

The 'metabolic barrier' is made up of enzymes which are mainly located in the peripheral processes of astrocytes. Drugs that can pass through the structural barrier may be metabolised by these enzymes before they reach the CNS. For example, ammonia and free fatty acids that can be potentially neurotoxic can freely cross the capillary endothelium but are metabolised before they reach the brain tissues.

Similarly, drugs such as ester local anaesthetics, dopamine, and norepinephrine are metabolised by monoamine oxidase and cholinesterase present in the capillary endothelium.

What type of drugs can easily pass through the blood–brain barrier?
Lower molecular weight, lipid soluble, unionised and protein unbound fractions of a drug can easily pass through blood–brain barrier. Some metabolic substrates – glucose and hormones like insulin and thyroxine can cross the barrier by carrier transport or endocytosis.

Name the parts of the brain that lie outside blood–brain barrier.
Choroid plexus, **A**rea postrema, **M**edian eminence and the **P**ineal gland (mnemonic: CAMP) lie outside the barrier.

Can you give some pathological conditions in which the blood–brain barrier is disrupted?
The integrity is impaired in inflammation, oedema, acute and chronic hypertension.

Write down the Henderson–Hasselbach equation for me.

$$pH = pK + \log [\text{conjugate base}]/[\text{acid}]$$

What is pKa?
pKa is the negative logarithm of the dissociation constant K. It is the pH at which the concerned chemical is half ionised and half unionised.

Why is it important to know about ionisation and the pKa of drugs?
Highly ionised drugs cannot cross lipid membranes whereas unionised drugs can cross freely. The unionised portion of a drug is the active portion. Morphine is highly ionised (76%), alfentanil is only 11% ionised (at pH of 7.4). Consequently the latter has a faster onset of action. The degree of ionisation depends on the pKa of the drug and the pH of the local environment. The pKa is the pH at which the drug is 50% ionised. Most drugs are either weak acids or weak bases. Acids are ionised in an alkaline environment and bases are ionised in an acidic environment.

The knowledge of this property of the drugs can be used to manipulate parameters such as onset of action and elimination. Local anaesthetics are weak bases. The closer the pKa of the local anaesthetic to the local tissue pH, the more unionised the drug is. That is why lidocaine (pKa 7.7) has a faster onset of action than bupivacaine (pKa 8.3). If the local tissues are alkalinised (e.g. by adding bicarbonate to the local anaesthetic), then the tissue pH is brought closer to the pKa, and the onset of action is hastened.

The rate of elimination of acidic drugs such as salicylates and barbiturates can be enhanced by alkalinisation of the urine. Similarly acid diuresis may be used in treatment of poisoning with basic drugs such as amphetamines.

What is ion trapping?
During pregnancy, weak bases like local anaesthetics and opioids that are unionised in physiological pH can easily cross placenta to enter the fetus. Fetal physiological pH is relatively acidic (7.2) and can be more acidic in fetal distress. In this circumstance these week bases gets converted to ionised form in the acidic environment. As the ionised form of the drug is lipid insoluble and cannot cross biological membranes, the drugs get 'trapped' in the fetus. This phenomenon is called ion trapping.

Q3 Anticholinesterases

Can you classify anticholinesterase drugs?
These drugs can broadly be classified into:

- Reversible:
  - Edrophonium.
  - Carbamate esters (e.g. neostigmine).
- Irreversible:
  - Organophosphorus compounds.

List some clinical uses of anticholinesterase drugs.

- To reverse the effect of non-depolarising muscle relaxants (e.g. neostigmine).
- In treatment of myasthenia gravis (e.g. pyridostigmine).
- Test to differentiate myasthenic crisis and cholinergic crisis in myasthenia gravis (e.g. edrophonium).
- Paralytic ileus and urinary retention (e.g. distigmine).
- Supraventricular tachycardia (e.g. neostigmine).

Can you briefly describe the structure of these anticholinesterase drugs and describe how they act?
Acetyl cholinesterase (AChE) basically contains two sites for binding an anionic site and esteratic site.

Edrophonium is a quaternary amine. The quaternary amine group attaches to the anionic site of AChE and hydrogen bonding occurs at the esteratic site. This is a readily reversible complex.

Carbamate esters can be tertiary or quaternary amines. The amine group attaches to the anionic site of AChE and the carbamyl group combines at the esteratic site. The complex is reversible and is subsequently hydrolysed.

Organophosphorus compounds causes phosphorylation of the esteratic site of AChE. The complex is extremely stable and is resistant to hydrolysis.

How does physostigmine differ from other carbamate esters?

Physostigmine is a tertiary amine. Neostigmine and pyridostigmine are quaternary amines that do not freely cross biological membranes. Physostigmine crosses biological membranes. When given orally it is well absorbed, penetrates cellular membranes, crosses the placenta and blood–brain barrier. Because of its ability to cross blood–brain barrier it has been used in the treatment of central anticholinergic syndrome caused by drugs with anticholinergic effects like atropine, tricyclic antidepressants but is no longer available.

What are the unwanted effects of anticholinesterases?

Although these drugs are commonly used to increase the local concentration of acetyl choline in the neuromuscular junction (nicotinic receptors) and improve neuromuscular transmission, they also have effects on the autonomic nervous system (muscarinic receptors) due to acetyl choline excess. The effects include:

- *Cardiovascular system*: Bradycardia, reduced cardiac output.
- *Central nervous system*: Miosis, blurred vision, central hypotensive effect.
- *Gastrointestinal tract*: Increase in tone and peristalsis can predispose to anastamotic breakdown following intestinal surgery, increased salivation.
- *Respiratory system*: Bronchoconstriction.
- *Neuromuscular junction*: High levels of neostigmine at the neuromuscular junction can directly block acetyl choline receptors. High-local concentrations of acetyl choline in the junction due to neostigmine can also cause a depolarising type of neuromuscular block.
- *Secretions*: In general all the secretions are increased – salivation, lacrimation, bronchorrhoea, diarrhoea.

Tell me about organophosphorus compound poisoning.

Organophosphorus compounds are readily absorbed by the lungs, skin and after oral ingestion. Organophosphorus compound poisoning is a well-known entity with numerous toxic manifestations including:

- *Nicotinic effects*: Muscle weakness and paralysis.
- *Muscarinic effects*: Increased secretions, increased smooth muscle tone, bradycardia.
- *Central effects*: Excitation, convulsion, tremors, coma and respiratory paralysis.

How would you treat organophosphorus compound poisoning?

- Airway, Breathing, Circulation.
- Ventilatory support, anticonvulsants.
- Repeated administration of atropine to treat muscarinic toxic effects.

- Acetyl choline reactivators such as pralidoxime which promotes hydrolysis of the phosphorylated AChE enzyme.

Clinical 6

Key topics: hypertension, laparoscopy, ventricular fibrillation, defibrillation, premedication

Q1 A 48-year-old female is listed for elective laparoscopic cholecystectomy. The student nurse on the ward bleeps you to tell that her blood pressure is 170/104 mmHg.

How will you proceed with this patient?

Go to the ward to see the patient in person. Thorough pre-anaesthetic assessment with special relevance to her blood pressure. Ensure that a correct size cuff is used and measure her blood pressure again.

The blood pressure is still high. What are you going to do?

History, examination, investigation.

Find out whether the patient is a known hypertensive; symptoms pertaining to cardiovascular disorders; other concurrent diseases like peripheral vascular disease, renal disease, cerebrovascular disease and diabetes mellitus that can be associated with high-blood pressure; medication the patient is taking.

General examination and specific system examination as directed by the history.

Investigations should include routine tests – full blood count, serum glucose (diabetes), urea, creatinine and electrolytes (renal impairment), electrocardiogram (left ventricular hypertrophy, ischaemic heart disease). If the history and examination findings are suggestive of any target organ dysfunction then further investigations such as a chest X-ray will be needed for thorough evaluation.

What could be the cause for high-blood pressure?

- Anxiety ('white coat hypertension').
- Essential (primary) hypertension.
- Secondary hypertension.

What options are available if you think it is due to anxiety?

- A sympathetic approach, explanation and reassurance often help more than medication.

- Anxiolytics (temazepam 20 mg orally) can be helpful.
- The operating list order can be rearranged in order to facilitate re-evaluation of the patient later.

Okay, the blood pressure still remains high in spite of reassurance and anxiolytics. She is not a known hypertensive. What are you going to do?

Discuss with a senior anaesthetist and the surgeon about the urgency of the surgery. Ideally the surgery needs to be postponed. The patient should be referred to her general practitioner for evaluation and control of blood pressure. Once the pressure is controlled then she can be re-listed for surgery after 4–6 weeks.

Why are you concerned about her hypertension?

Hypertensive patients have increased vascular reactivity. Depending on the chronicity of the condition they could have developed smooth muscle hypertrophy in the arterioles as well as left ventricular hypertrophy due to increased strain on the heart. As a result, for a given change in the sympathetic nervous system activity the blood pressure changes are much exaggerated. Laparoscopic procedure involves significant hemodynamic disturbance.

Hypertension can be associated with other diseases of relevance to anaesthesia such as ischaemic heart disease, peripheral vascular disease, cerebrovascular disease, renal disease and diabetes mellitus. These patients have an increased risk of adverse perioperative cardiac events.

Why should you wait for 4–6 weeks, why not anaesthetise her after controlling her blood pressure immediately with anti-hypertensives?

Blood pressure can be acutely controlled, but the vascular reactivity still persists. The exaggerated swings in the blood pressure are lessened in controlled hypertension.

How does hypertension affect myocardial oxygen supply/demand balance?

In hypertensive patients the systemic vascular resistance is high. This increases the afterload to the heart. In the long run due to the strain to the left heart there is left ventricular hypertrophy. Both these factors increase myocardial oxygen demand.

Coronary perfusion pressure is aortic diastolic pressure minus left ventricular end-diastolic pressure (LVEDP). Increased LVEDP in hypertensive patients decreases effective coronary perfusion in susceptible areas thereby predisposing to subendocardial ischemia.

What is the relevance of degree of hypertension to anaesthesia?

Table 6.2 *Relevance of degree of hypertension to anaesthesia*

Degree of hypertension	Diastolic pressure (mmHg)	Prognosis with anaesthesia
Mild	90–104	No evidence that treatment makes any difference to outcome
Moderate	105–114	Not really looked at but presumably increased risk, particularly if evidence of end organ damage
Severe	>114	Probably increased risk of ischaemia, arrhythmia and poor outcome therefore cancel and treat

What are the anaesthetic implications of laparoscopic cholecystectomy?

The specific challenges in managing patients for laparoscopic cholecystectomy are those due to:

- Positioning.
- Insufflation.
- Instrumentation.
- Environment.

Laparoscopic cholecystectomy offers the advantage of early ambulation and faster recovery but the physiological insult intraoperatively can be greater than the open procedure.

Why is positioning a patient important and what precautions will you take in positioning any patient?

Positioning a patient is done to improve surgical access. Care should be taken while positioning as there are hazards associated with pressure and physiological changes.

Pressure can cause undue compression on pressure points on skin, tendon and joints or on nerves. Physiological changes are mainly associated with gravitationally dictated venous pooling and effects on venous return. In the respiratory system, depending on the position, functional residual capacity (FRC) and total lung volume can be affected.

Other than the pressure and physiological changes, care should be taken to avoid accidental dislodgement or displacement of intra venous access, airway, monitoring, etc.

What are the problems due to instrumentation in laparoscopy?

Inadvertent damage to major vessels can lead to massive bleeding. Peritoneal stretching can lead to severe vagal bradycardia. There is a risk of laparoscopic procedures getting converted to open procedures if the anatomy is difficult.

What are the effects of insufflation of abdominal cavity?

The effects are due to mechanical compression and systemic absorption of carbon dioxide.

- *Mechanical compression*: The abdomen is filled to high pressure with carbon dioxide which results in:
  - *Cardiovascular system*: Decreased venous return, increased systemic resistance, mechanical distortion of the position of the heart, decreased cardiac output and possibility of air embolism.
  - *Respiratory system*: Splinting of diaphragm, compression on lungs, reduced FRC and shunting of blood. Carina can get widened and trachea can move up resulting in endobronchial intubation. Possibility of pneumothorax.
  - *Gastrointestinal tract*: Increased intragastric pressure encouraging regurgitation. Stretching of peritoneum can cause bradycardia.
- *Systemic absorption*: Absorption of carbon dioxide increases PCO_2 causing acidosis, right shift of the oxygen dissociation curve and hypertension. Controlled ventilation intraoperatively can be helpful to negate these effects to an extent.

Are there any maximal safe limits for insufflation?

The recommended maximum intraperitoneal pressure is 20 cmH_2O. This can be achieved most of the time when the administered gas flow does not exceed 4 l/min and the intraperitoneal gas volume does not exceed 3–5 l.

How will you manage post-operative pain in this patient?

Local anaesthetic infiltration at the site of the wounds. Combination of simple analgesics, paracetamol and non-steroidal anti-inflammatory drugs (NSAIDs) along with 'as required' opioids is usually sufficient. The main advantage of the laparoscopic procedure is its faster recovery and minimal tissue handling.

During the immediate recovery period patients can complain of shoulder pain due to diaphragmatic irritation and residual pneumoperitoneum. Laparoscopic procedures are notorious in causing severe post-operative nausea and vomiting (PONV). Controlling PONV with multimodal approach is important as PONV and post-operative pain can compound each other.

Q2 Critical incident: ventricular fibrillation

Alright. Now consider that the patient is on the operating table, halfway through a laparoscopic cholecystectomy. You notice that there are frequent ventricular ectopics on the monitor. What will you do?

- Check Airway, Breathing, Circulation.
- Are the ectopics causing haemodynamic disturbance? Look for possible causes:
  - *Patient factors*: Electrolyte disturbance, ischaemic heart disease.

- *Anaesthetic factors*: Hypoxia, hypercarbia, hypotension.
- *Surgical factors*: Insufflation, instrumentation.

As you are looking for the causes of these ectopics you observe that the ectopics become more frequent and the ECG turns to this rhythm:

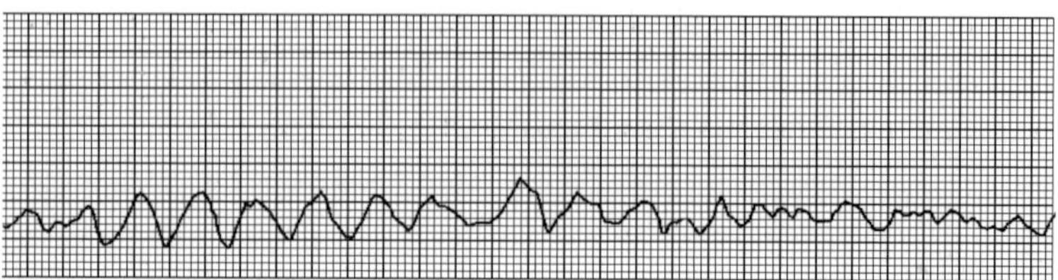

Figure 6.5 *Ventricular Fibrillation*

What will you do now?

ECG shows ventricular fibrillation:

- Call for senior help.
- Tell surgeon to stop surgery and deflate.
- Check electrodes, confirm ventricular fibrillation.
- Advanced Life Support algorithm – cardio-pulmonary resuscitation (CPR).
- Defibrillation × 3 times (200–200–360 J).
- Epinephrine 1 mg every 3 min.
- Defibrillation 360–360–360 J.
- Continue CPR.
- Recheck Airway, Breathing, Circulation.
- Check electrodes, consider amiodarone, buffers.
- Look for a treatable cause.

What are the potentially reversible causes?

Hypoxia, hypovolaemia, hypo/hyperkalaemia, hypothermia.

Tension pneumothorax, toxic/therapeutic disorders, tamponade, thromboembolic and mechanical obstruction.

What factors affect successful defibrillation?

- *Transthoracic impedance*: It is influenced by electrode or paddle size, the paddle-skin coupling material, number and time interval of previous shocks, phase of ventilation, distance between the electrodes and paddle pressure.

  The standard adult paddle size is 13 cm in diameter; the paddle-skin coupling material is either liquid gel or semisolid gel pads; shocks administered in close sequence can reduce the subsequent impedance; impedance is less when lung volume is less – after expiratory phase; applying firm paddle pressure of about 10 kg force helps in maintaining good skin contact and reducing impedance.

- *Shock energy*: Excessive current delivered to myocardium can damage it. Initial two shocks should be 200 J. Only when it is ineffective escalate to 360 J.
- *Biphasic defibrillation*: Superior to monophasic defibrillation. Successful biphasic defibrillation requires less energy.
- *Electrode position*: This should allow maximum current flow through myocardium. Though anterior–posterior placing of electrodes is more effective, it is easier to place one electrode to the right of upper sternum below clavicle and other one in the fifth intercostal space in the anterior axillary line.

Q3 Premedication

Tell me about the ASA scoring system.

The ASA scoring system (American Society of Anesthesiologists) describes the preoperative condition of a patient and is used routinely for every patient in the UK. It makes no allowances for the patient's age, smoking history, obesity or pregnancy. Anticipated difficulties in intubation are not relevant. Addition of the postscript E indicates emergency surgery. There is some correlation between ASA score and peri-operative mortality. Definitions applied in the ASA system are as follows (peri-operative mortality in brackets):

I: Healthy patient (0.1%)
II: Mild systemic disease, no functional limitation (0.2%)
III: Moderate systemic disease, definite functional limitation (1.8%)
IV: Severe systemic disease that is a constant threat to life (7.8%)
V: Moribund patient, unlikely to survive 24 hours with or without operation (9.4%)

A sixth category has been added to refer to a brain-dead patient who is to undergo organ harvest (and who is therefore definitely going to have 100% mortality).

What are the indications for premedication of patients?

As more day surgery is performed and more patients are admitted to hospital close to the scheduled time of surgery, premedication has become less common. The main indication for premedication remains anxiety, for which a benzodiazepine is usually prescribed, sometimes with metoclopramide to promote absorption. Premedication serves several purposes:

- Anxiolysis.
- Smoother induction of anaesthesia.
- Reduced requirement for intravenous induction agents.
- Reduced likelihood of awareness.
- Reduced aspiration risk.
- Analgesia.

Intramuscular opioids are now rarely prescribed as premedication. The prevention of aspiration pneumonitis in patients with reflux requires premedication with an H_2-antagonist, the evening before and morning of surgery, and sodium citrate administration immediately prior to induction of anaesthesia. Topical local anaesthetic cream over two potential sites for venous cannulation is usually prescribed for children. Anticholinergic agents may be prescribed to dry secretions or to prevent bradycardia (e.g. during squint surgery). Usual medication should be continued up to the time of anaesthesia.

Specific advantages of anti-sialagogues relate to bronchoscopic procedures where reduced secretions aid the ease with which the procedure can be carried out. Such premedication is also of use when ketamine is to be given (due to its effect on increasing salivary and bronchial secretions).

Overall, explanation of the process of anaesthesia to patients has greatly reduced the need for sedative and anxiolytic premedicants – all of which may delay recovery in the early period.

Other than in exceptional circumstances (extreme nervousness or hospital phobia) sedative premedication is not used in day-case patients.

There is a vogue for pre-operative administration of analgesics as a type of premedication. Paracetamol and non-steroidal anti-inflammatory drugs (NSAIDs) have been used in this way, either by oral or rectal use. Diclofenac suppositories are in widespread usage for this purpose. Administration must be explained to the patient (and consent obtained).

Physics, clinical measurement and safety 6

Key topics: intracranial pressure monitoring, pulse oximetry, ultrasound

Q1 Intracranial pressure monitoring

What are the indications for monitoring intracranial pressure (ICP)?

ICP monitoring is indicated in patients with severe head injury, post-operative monitoring following major intracranial surgery in the intensive care unit and in patients with any cause of coma and raised ICP. The threshold to monitor ICP invasively varies between units.

How do you monitor ICP?

Clinically, serial neurological examination to monitor for raised ICP. These include Glasgow Coma Scale, vital parameters (*Cushing's reflex*: increase in mean arterial pressure and decrease in heart rate), pupillary signs and focal neurological signs.

Radiological investigations such as computerised tomography scan can be useful to find the markers for increased ICP like midline shift, obliteration of ventricles, etc.

ICP can be continuously monitored using two different systems:

1 Fibreoptic probes,
2 Pressure transducers.

Can you tell me more about continuous monitoring equipment?

A fibreoptic probe is usually placed epidurally. Using a burr hole the probe is placed between skull and dura. This mode of monitoring is less reliable than the pressure transducer systems but has the advantage of being technically easier with low-infection rates. Fibreoptic probes can also be placed inside the ventricles.

A direct type of pressure transducer systems can be placed in:

- Subarachnoid space.
- Ventricles.
- Intraparenchyma.

In the subarachnoid space a subarachnoid bolt is applied via a burr hole. The accuracy is more reliable but this carries a high-infection rate.

Ventricular drains are generally placed intraoperatively under direct vision. In this situation, apart from monitoring the ICP, it also provides an access for therapeutic drainage of cerebrospinal fluid if needed. This method of ICP monitoring carries the highest rate for infection.

The intraparenchymal or intracerebral transducer is placed directly within the brain tissue.

How do these systems work?

The fibreoptic device consists of two light paths. One carries light to the tip of the catheter, the other returns reflected light from the tip. The amount of light returned depends on the angle of reflecting surface at the tip which in turn depends on the pressure within.

In the direct pressure transducer devices ICP waves are transmitted via a fluid filled tube to a strain-gauge transducer. Waveforms and digital readings are displayed on the monitor.

How can you describe the waveform obtained in the ICP monitors?

The skull being a rigid box, the three components that contribute to the ICP are blood, CSF and brain. The pressure changes in the blood are more dynamic than that in CSF or brain. Therefore the ICP waveform mostly resembles the arterial waveform. Factors affecting central venous pressure (CVP) like respiration and cough can also affect the waveform.

What is the normal ICP?

Under resting conditions, in supine position, the mean ICP varies between 7 and 15 mmHg.

Q2 Pulse oximetry

What are the basic principles of pulse oximetry?

Pulse oximetry works based on spectrophotometry. The principles can be described by the Beer–Lambert law. Beer's law concerns the concentration of the substance involved and Lambert's law concerns the thickness of the substance involved.

- *Beer's law*: Intensity of transmitted light decreases exponentially as the concentration of the substance increases.
- *Lambert's law*: Intensity of the transmitted light decreases exponentially as the distance travelled through the substance increases.

Combining both the laws states that the amount of light absorbed by the solution is directly proportional to the molar concentration and thickness of the solution.

Can you tell me how the pulse oximeter works?

Oximetry is a photometric technique that measures percentage haemoglobin saturation. The light absorbed by blood depends on the quantities of deoxyhaemoglobin and oxyhaemoglobin present and the wavelength of the light.

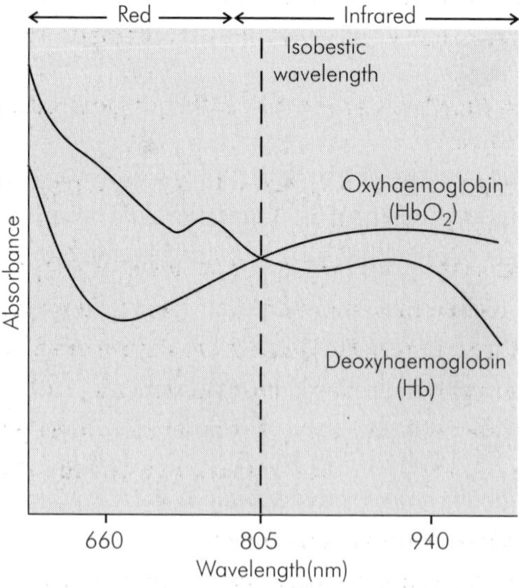

Figure 6.6 *Absorbance curves in oximetry*

The probe consists of two light emitting diodes, one emits light at 660 nm wavelength (red region) and other emits at 940 nm wave length (infra-red region). The diodes are switched on and off with a pause several hundred times a second. The other side of the pulse oximeter probe has a photodetector. The output of the sensors is processed electronically to give a pulse waveform and the arterial oxygen saturation.

Deoxyhaemoglobin absorbs maximum light at red region (660 nm wavelength). At 940 nm absorbance of oxyhaemoglobin is greater than deoxyhaemoglobin. There is a microprocessor with an inbuilt algorithm in which the ratio of absorption at red region to infrared region (R/IR) corresponds to an empirically found saturation value.

The light absorbed by the arterial blood is variable due to the pulsatile flow. Light absorbed by skin, soft tissues, bone, non-pulsatile component of arterial blood and venous blood is constant. The microprocessor also differentiates pulsatile flow from that of non-pulsatile flow.

Why are the diodes switched on and off in sequence with a pause?
During the pause period it can detect the ambient light and compensate for it.

How do the manufacturers pre-calibrate pulseoximeters?
Oximeters were calibrated using previously obtained data from human volunteer studies, in which the saturations were recorded while subjects breathed various inspired oxygen concentrations including hypoxic levels. On ethical grounds these studies were limited to minimum measured saturations of 85%. Normalised R/IR ratio is measured using photoplethysmography and at the same time blood saturation values were obtained directly from a standard in vitro oximeter. Hence a graph with relationship between R/IR ratio and SaO_2 is obtained.

What is the response time for desaturation with a finger probe? What factors affect the response time?
Pulse oximeters average their reading every 10–20 s. The response time for desaturation with a finger probe is more than 60 s.

Two factors can affect the response time. Instrumental delay is related to the averaging time used to reduce movement artifact. Prolonged averaging time prolongs the response time. Circulatory delay is due to the time taken for changes in the central saturation to reach the periphery and this depends on the site of the probe. Response time is shorter with ear probe as compared to finger probe. Both vasoconstriction and venous engorgement can increase response time by 2–3-fold.

What are the limitations of the pulse oximetry?

- Pulse oximeter readings are not accurate in the presence of abnormal haemoglobins. Carboxyhaemoglobin has similar absorbance to oxyhaemoglobin at

660 nm, hence it overestimates the saturation. In methaemoglobinaemia at high saturations the true value is underestimated; at low saturations it is overestimated.

- Pulse oximeters are less accurate at low haemoglobin levels (below 8 g/dl).
- Dyes such as methylene blue leads to a falsely low reading.
- High-frequency radio-interference from diathermy can affect some pulse oximeter readings. The effect can be reduced by using suppression filters.
- Vasoconstriction, low-cardiac output and reduced peripheral circulation can lead to inaccuracy in the reading.
- The effect of ambient light is minimised using shielded probes and sequential light emitting diode (LED) cycling. Bright external lights can affect performance.
- Motion artefacts such as shivering or seizure activity can result in inaccurate reading. These artefacts can be reduced by increasing the signal averaging time.

What is a co-oximeter? How does it differ from pulse oximeter?

A co-oximeter is a spectrophotometer that uses four different wavelengths and hence it can measure total haemoglobin, oxyhaemoglobin, carboxyhaemoglobin and methaemoglobin. Pulse oximeters use only two wavelengths. Co-oximeters are incorporated into blood gas analysers. They are not suitable to provide continuous saturation monitoring.

Q3 Ultrasound

What is ultrasound?

It is a high-frequency sound wave above the range of human hearing (>20,000 Hz). A sound wave of 3–15 MHz is produced by medical ultrasound devices.

How does ultrasound based equipment work?

Ultrasound relies on the transmission if high-frequency vibrations and detection of the reflected signals from tissue interfaces.

An ultrasound wave of a known frequency is passed through the tissues. Some of it is absorbed by the tissues and part of it is reflected off the boundaries and tissue interfaces. The amount of ultrasound reflected depends on the tissue interface concerned (vessel wall and blood or fluid). The difference between the transmitted and reflected sound wave helps to identify various structures and objects. It mainly helps to identify the boundaries between the structures where there is change in the tissue interface.

What is in the ultrasound probe?
It contains a transducer and piezoelectric crystal.

What does the transducer do?
It converts one form of energy in to another. Here the electrical energy is converted into sound waves. The returned sound waves are then converted back into an electrical signal.

Can you tell me how ultrasound waves are generated?
A voltage is applied to the crystal. The change in the shape of the crystal generates oscillations which are propagated as ultrasound waves.

Why do we use gel on the probe?
Air is very poor transmitter of ultrasound. It reflects most of the ultrasound and very little is transmitted to the tissues. This hurdle is eliminated by applying conducting gels.

What other substances reflect ultrasound?
Other than gas, bones and fat can reflect ultrasound and appear white on screen. Also needles and probes used for various interventions can be identified as 'white images' as they do not transmit ultrasound.

Tell me about the principle used in Doppler.
The Doppler principle is based on the property of a change in the frequency of the reflected signals from moving objects.

The difference between the emitted and reflected frequency (frequency shift) is directly proportional to the speed of movement (velocity). The flow rate can be calculated by estimating the cross sectional area of the vessel and integrating it with the velocity.

What are the clinical applications of ultrasound and Doppler?
Ultrasound and Doppler can be used in diagnostic purposes or to assist some therapeutic interventions:
- Echocardiography.
- Fetal imaging.
- Localisation of central veins for cannulation.
- Ultrasound guided nerve blocks.

- Assessing epidural space depth in paediatrics.
- Diagnostic applications in intra-abdominal, pelvic and thoracic pathologies.
- Assisting insertion of pleural drains.

Ultrasound uses the Doppler principle and analysis of the reflected frequencies allows determination of velocity of flow. This is used in transcranial Doppler, fetal blood flow monitoring, Doppler plethysmography and in cardiac output measurements such as trans-oesophageal Doppler.

SOE 7

Physiology 7

Key topics: renal physiology, exercise, neuromuscular junction

Q1 Renal physiology: renal blood flow/glomerular filtration rate

What is the normal renal blood flow (RBF)? How is it distributed?

The kidneys receive 1000–1250 ml of blood per minute, which is 20–25% of total cardiac output. The renal cortex gets about 500 ml/min/100 g. The outer medulla receives 100 ml/min/100 g and the inner medulla receives 200 ml/min/100 g.

Can you describe in detail the arrangement of blood vessels in the kidney?

Renal artery → Interlobar artery → Arcuate arteries → Interlobular arteries → Afferent arterioles.

The renal artery is a direct branch of aorta that enters the kidney at the hilum. It branches to form interlobar arteries, which in turn branch to form arcuate arteries. As the name implies arcuate arteries have a curved course and run along the boundary between the cortex and medulla. The interlobular arteries branch at right angles from the arcuate arteries from which the afferent arterioles finally emerge.

The glomerulus contains a tuft of capillaries. These capillaries are unique in that they originate from arterioles and also drain to arterioles.

The efferent arterioles branch to form the peritubular capillaries that surround the tubules. They also give rise to vasa recta, which play an important role in countercurrent exchange.

The capillaries drain into the renal vein, which leaves the hilum of kidney.

What do you mean by autoregulation? How does it work in the kidneys?

Autoregulation is a protective property of organs to maintain blood flow over a wide range of blood pressures. The proposed theories for autoregulation include:

- *Myogenic theory* – whereby an increase in the wall tension of blood vessels produced by increased perfusion pressure causes reflex contraction of smooth muscles in the vessel wall.
- *Metabolic theory* – where local blood supply is regulated by the local presence of metabolic end products.

In the kidney this autoregulation works within a range of mean arterial pressures of 90–200 mmHg.

What is the normal glomerular filtration rate (GFR) and what factors determine the filtration?

The GFR is about 125 ml/min (180 l/day). Broadly, two factors determine filtration:

- The molecules involved.
- Glomerular filtration forces.

With regard to molecules, size is the main determinant. Smaller molecules with a size less than 7000 Da are freely filtered and the cut-off molecular weight is about 70,000. The other important determinant is the charge of molecules. Glomerular basement membrane has heparan sulphate proteoglycan and the foot processes contain sialoglycoproteins. Both are negatively charged and hence both repel negatively charged molecules like albumin and interrupt filtration.

In respect of glomerular filtration forces, GFR is proportional to the forces that favours filtration minus the forces that opposes the filtration, that is:

$$\text{GFR} \propto (P_G + \pi_B) - (P_B + \pi_G)$$

where P_G = Hydrostatic pressure in glomerular capillaries, P_B = Hydrostatic pressure in Bowman's capsule, π_B = Colloid osmotic pressure in Bowman's capsule and π_G = Colloid osmotic pressure in glomerular capillaries.

The glomerular capillaries are unique in that they start from an arteriole and end in another arteriole. Due to the high-pressure system at both ends their hydrostatic pressure is 45 mmHg, which is considerably higher than the 32 mmHg in other capillary beds. The permeability of glomerular capillaries is about 100 times greater than the permeability of capillaries in the rest of the body.

What do you mean by the term 'filtration fraction'?

Filtration fraction is the fraction of renal plasma flow (RPF) filtered in the glomerulus. The RBF is about 1100 ml/min. Of this 600 ml is plasma and the rest constitutes the red cells, which are not filtered. RPF is 600 ml/min and the GFR is 120 ml/min. Thus the filtration fraction is 120/600 ml (i.e. about 20%).

What is tubulo-glomerular feedback?

Tubulo-glomerular feedback is a mechanism whereby the single nephron GFR is adjusted by a feedback mechanism determined by the characteristic of the tubular fluid. This is a protective mechanism to maintain the GFR to match the reabsorptive capacity of individual nephrons.

How can you measure GFR and RPF?

These are indirectly measured by measuring the renal clearances of certain substances. The clearance of a substance is given by the formula C = UV/P where C is the clearance of the substance, U and P are the urine and plasma concentration, respectively and V is the urine flow in ml/min.

Inulin clearance is used for the measurement of GFR. It has a relatively small molecular weight of 5500 Da and is therefore freely filtered in the glomerulus. It is not reabsorbed, secreted, metabolised nor synthesised in kidney. Therefore it represents the GFR.

Para amino hippuric acid (PAH) is used to measure RPF. It is not only freely filtered in glomerulus but is also secreted by proximal tubule. Therefore it represents the RPF.

Is there any alternative, more practical way of measuring GFR?

Creatinine clearance is an alternative way to measure GFR. Unlike inulin, which is an exogenous substance, creatinine is a product of muscle metabolism. It is freely filtered in the glomerulus but not affected by tubular reabsorption, metabolism or synthesis. Although to a small extent it is secreted in the tubules, it gives a reasonable estimate of GFR.

How will you calculate RBF from RPF?

Blood has a composition of 45% haematocrit and 55% plasma. Therefore the measure of RPF represents 55% of the RBF. The RBF can be calculated by the formula,

$$\text{RBF} = \text{RPF} \times 100/55.$$

Q2 Physiology of exercise

Can you tell me about the physiological changes occurring during unaccustomed exercise?

Physiological changes can be grossly divided into two – central changes and regional changes. Anticipation of activity increases sympathetic discharge and inhibits parasympathetic discharge. There is cerebrocortical activation of the sympathetic system as impulses from muscle mechanoreceptors activate cardiovascular reflexes and baroreceptor reflexes come into play. At regional level, local reflexes are stimulated by the accumulation of metabolites.

What happens to regional blood flow?

Blood flow is diverted to active skeletal muscles from the kidneys, splanchnic region and inactive muscles. Cutaneous blood flow is decreased initially and increased later due to rising body temperature and in severe exercise it decreases again due to cutaneous vasoconstriction when the oxygen extraction in the muscle increases enormously. Cerebral blood flow is unaltered and the myocardial blood flow increases to meet the metabolic demand.

What is the normal resting blood flow to skeletal muscles?

It is very low, 2–4 ml/100 g/min. (about 1200 ml/min). This can increase up to 10 times during exercise.

What mechanisms are involved in increasing the blood flow to skeletal muscle?

Increase in PCO_2, decrease in PO_2, accumulation of adenosine, potassium and acidosis all lead to local vasodilatation. Acidosis, increase in 2,3-diphosphoglycerate (DPG) and rising temperature, shift the oxygen dissociation curve to the right.

What cardiovascular changes occur during exercise?

Increased sympathetic activity and decreased parasympathetic activity result in increased heart rate and cardiac output. Venous return is increased due to increased muscle activity, there is an increase in thoracic pump activity due to increased respiratory rate and tidal volume. Both systolic and diastolic blood pressures increase during exercise. Systolic pressure increases more than diastolic and as a result the pulse pressure is increased. Vasodilatation in active muscles results in decreased systemic vascular resistance.

What can happen when someone continues to exercise to the point of exhaustion?

The compensatory mechanisms fail to cope up with unaccustomed severe exercise beyond a limit. Heart rate rises to about 180 beats per minute and plateaus at that rate. Stroke volume starts decreasing and blood pressure drops. Excessive sympathetic activity causes profound vasoconstriction. Heat loss is not in par with heat production and hence body temperature rises. Accumulation of carbon dioxide and lactic acid leads to acidosis. Unbearable muscle cramps and pain ensue and the drive to continue the activity is lost.

Q3 Neuromuscular junction

Can you draw a diagram of a neuromuscular junction and describe the various components?

A neuromuscular junction typically comprises a motor nerve ending and a muscle motor end plate. There is a junctional gap between the two. As the myelinated motor

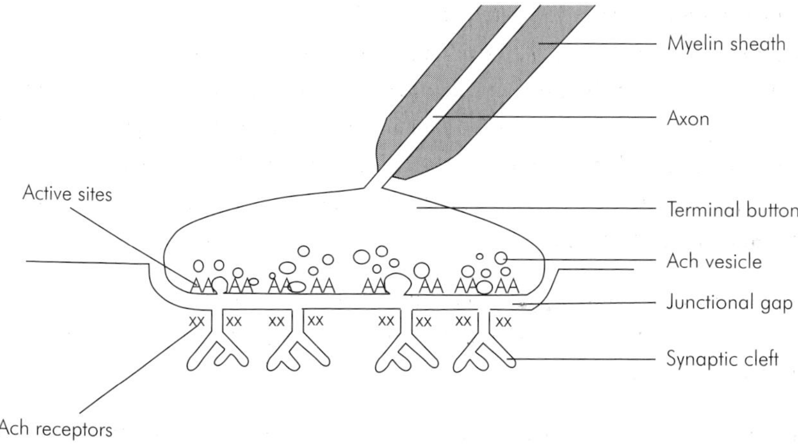

Figure 7.1 *Structure of the NMJ*

nerve reaches the muscle it becomes unmyelinated and undergoes branching. The corresponding adjacent muscle membrane gets thickened and invaginated to form junctional folds. The crest of the junctional folds contains the acetylcholine receptors. Generally there are about 50 million acetylcholine receptors in a motor end plate.

Tell me more about the acetylcholine receptors.

The acetylcholine receptor is of the nicotinic type. These proteins are made up of five subunits, two α, one β, one ε and one δ subunits. These five subunits are arranged around a central pore that is generally closed in the resting state. The two alpha subunits have specific binding sites for acetylcholine receptors. When acetylcholine molecules occupy both the binding sites the central pore opens and acts as an ionic channel for Na^+ ions.

Other than this junctional acetylcholine receptor what other nicotinic receptors are present in this area?

There are pre-junctional receptors located in the nerve terminals and extra-junctional receptors scattered in the muscle membrane.

Can you tell more about extra-junctional receptors?

Structurally, extra-junctional receptors are different from the junctional ones by having a γ subunit instead of ε subunit. Normally this is present during fetal life and in early neonates. As the neuromuscular transmission mechanism becomes well established these extra-junctional acetylcholine receptors gradually diminish in number. In pathological states (such as paraplegia) there is a proliferation of the extra-junctional receptors. In these circumstances if suxamethonium is used it can affect these extra-junctional receptors (that have a longer depolarisation time) resulting in massive extrusion of K^+ ions and life-threatening hyperkalaemia.

Describe the synthesis and storage of acetylcholine in the nerve terminal.

Acetylcholine is synthesised by a reaction between acetyl-CoA and choline. The reaction is catalysed by the enzyme choline acetyltransferase. Acetyl-CoA is in turn synthesised from pyruvate in the mitochondria of the axon terminals. Half of the choline is obtained from the extra-cellular fluid (this depends on an active process in the cell membrane which is the rate limiting step in the synthesis of acetylcholine) and the remaining half of the choline is derived from the breakdown of acetylcholine in the synaptic cleft. Choline acetyl transferase is synthesised from the cell bodies of the motor neurons and reaches the nerve terminal by axoplasmic flow:

$$\text{Acetyl-CoA} + \text{Choline} \xrightarrow{\text{(choline acetyl transferase)}} \text{Acetylcholine}$$

$$\text{Acetylcholine} \xrightarrow{\text{(acetylcholine esterases)}} \text{Choline} + \text{Acetate}$$

Once formed, acetylcholine molecules are stored in small vesicles in the nerve terminals. Most of the vesicles are close to the junction as a readily releasable store and about 20% of the vesicles remain as a stationary reserve.

What is a miniature end plate potential?

By a process described as 'exocytosis' the vesicles situated closer to the presynaptic membrane release their content spontaneously into the synaptic cleft in a random fashion. This released acetylcholine in the neuromuscular junction acts on the acetylcholine receptors to produce a small transient electrical response in the postsynaptic membrane described as miniature end plate potential.

What do you mean by 'margin of safety' with regards to neuromuscular transmission?

During neuromuscular transmission, each nerve impulse results in the release of about 60 vesicles from the nerve terminal into the junctional cleft. Each vesicle contains about 4000 molecules of acetylcholine. This amount of acetylcholine molecules is about 10 times more than that is actually needed for a normal neuromuscular transmission. This is the 'margin of safety'.

Pharmacology 7

Key topics: drug action, receptors, antiemetics, statistical tests

Q1 Drug action

Can you describe different ways or mechanisms by which drugs produce their effects?

Drugs may act in various ways to produce their effects. A single drug or a group of drugs often act by several mechanisms, at different target sites.

- Physiochemical, where drug activity is related to the physiochemical properties of the drug.
- Enzyme inhibition.
- Receptor activation.

Can you give some examples where clinical effects are due to the physiochemical properties of the drug?

Various physiochemical properties – osmolarity, pH, adsorption and chelation will result in clinical effects. For example:

- Mannitol when administered intravenously increases the plasma osmolarity and draws water from tissues and it produces osmotic diuresis.
- Antacids exert their effect by neutralising gastric acid.
- Activated charcoal has a large surface area for a given mass hence it is given orally to adsorb ingested poisons and drugs.
- Penicillamine is used as a chelating agent to treat metal poisoning.
- The mechanism of action of general anaesthetics can be explained by physiochemical properties such as lipid solubility and expansion of hydrophobic sites (critical volume expansion theory).

Can you give some examples for enzyme inhibition?

- Captopril inhibits angiotensin-converting enzyme (ACE inhibitor) and there by reduces the conversion of angiotensinogen I–II and acts as an anti-hypertensive agent.
- Neostigmine causes reversible inhibition of acetyl cholinesterase and therefore increases the concentration of acetylcholine.
- Non-steroidal anti-inflammatory drugs (NSAIDs) inhibit cyclo-oxygenase enzyme and produce an anti-inflammatory effect.

What is a receptor?

It is a protein molecule, usually located in the cell membrane which selectively binds with extra-cellular compounds (ligand). This binding results in biochemical events within the cell.

What are the types of receptors? Can you give examples for drugs acting on these receptors?

There are at least four types of receptors:

1 *Ligand-gated ion channels*: These receptors are located on the cell membrane. Examples include the nicotinic receptor (neuromuscular blocking drugs) and NMDA receptor (ketamine).
2 *Tyrosine-kinase-coupled receptors*: These are also located on the cell membrane. Examples are the insulin receptor and growth factor receptor.
3 *Intracellular receptors*: These are located inside the cells. This group includes the steroid receptor.
4 *G-protein-coupled receptors*: These span the cell membrane. Examples are opioid receptors and the adrenoreceptor.

What are the various mechanisms by which the receptor can initiate biochemical events?

When a ligand or drug binds to a receptor, the resulting receptor–ligand complex or receptor–drug complex produces the following changes:

- Direct changes in ionic permeability. For example, binding of acetylcholine to nicotinic receptor causes conformational change in the structure of the receptor and opens the ion channel. This results in influx of Na^+ ions. Benzodiazepines bind to GABA receptors ($GABA_A$), resulting in chloride influx to produce membrane hyperpolarisation.
- Accumulation of intermediate messengers (cAMP, cGMP). Epinephrine for example, binds to G-protein coupled receptors to increase the cyclic AMP. Cyclic AMP acts as an intermediate messenger in this situation.
- Regulation of gene transcription: Thyroid hormones and steroids alter the expression of DNA and RNA.

What are the characteristics of drug–receptor interaction?

The interaction of a drug with a receptor is specific, dose-related and saturable.

What are G-proteins?

These are regulatory proteins (GTP-binding proteins), which indirectly couple the receptor to adenylyl cyclase enzyme. They have a heterotrimeric structure (three different subunits, α, β and γ). G-protein stimulates (Gs) or inhibits (Gi) the activity of adenylyl cyclase and alters the synthesis of cAMP. G-proteins can produce considerable amplification of the biological stimulus produced by receptor occupation, because Gs (or Gi) can be repeatedly activated by a single agonist–receptor complex. Consequently many drugs acting on G-proteins are extremely potent.

Can you name the different types of G-proteins?

G-proteins are of various types – Gs, Gi, Gq, Gr (in retina) and Gt (in nose). Gq-protein controls the receptor-mediated activation of phospholipase C and breakdown of phosphoinositides.

Can you give me some examples of receptor G-protein interactions?

Opioids and α_2-adrenergic agonists interact with Gi-proteins to reduce the activity of adenylyl cyclase and this results in reduced neurotransmission.

β_1-adrenergic agonists interact with Gs-proteins and increase the activity of adenylyl cyclase results in increased levels of cAMP and increased cardiac contraction.

α_1-adrenergic agonists bind to Gq-proteins and activate phospholipase C which results in increased production of inositol triphosphate and diacylglycerol (DAG).

What are the different types of histamine receptors?

- H_1 receptors are responsible for smooth muscle contraction in the gastro-intestinal tract, uterus and bronchi. Vascular smooth muscle relaxes, with increased vascular permeability. There is also stimulation and irritation of cutaneous nerve endings.
- H_2 receptor stimulation causes production of acid, pepsin and intrinsic factor secretion from gastric mucosa.
- H_3 receptors are present in brain and thought to inhibit histamine release.
- H_4 receptors are identified only experimentally.

Q2 Anti-emetic drugs

What are the various receptors involved in the mechanism of nausea and vomiting?

There are many receptors and neural pathways involved in nausea and vomiting. They include histamine (H_1), dopamine (D_2), muscarinic (M_3), serotonin ($5HT_3$) and neurokinin (NK) receptors. Other receptors such as opioid receptors also have a role. These receptors are located in the chemoreceptor trigger zone in the area postrema, vomiting centre in medulla and some are located peripherally in the GIT.

- Dopamine receptors are located in the area postrema (chemoreceptor trigger zone). They are also present in the nucleus of tractus solitarius and dorsal motor vagal nucleus.

- 5-hydroxytryptamine (5-HT_3) receptors are distributed centrally in the area postrema, nucleus tractus solitarius, cerebral cortex and hippocampus and peripherally in the gut mucosa.
- Acetylcholine receptors are found in the nucleus tractus solitarius and dorsal motor vagal nucleus.
- Histamine receptors are concentrated in the nucleus tractus solitarius and dorsal motor vagal nucleus.
- Opioid receptors are situated in the area postrema and when stimulated cause vomiting.
- NK receptors are widely distributed in both central and peripheral nervous systems.

Classify drugs used for control of nausea and vomiting.

- Dopamine antagonists:
  - Phenothiazines (chlorpromazine, prochlorperazine).
  - Butyrophenones (droperidol, domperidone).
  - Benzamides (metoclopramide).
- Anticholinergics (hyoscine).
- Antihistamines (cyclizine, promethazine).
- 5-HT_3 antagonists (ondansetron, granisetron).
- Miscellaneous (steroids, canabinoids, lorazepam, propofol, acupuncture).

How does ondansetron work?

Ondansetron is a competitive, highly selective antagonist of 5-HT_3 (serotonin) subtype 3 receptors. 5-HT_3 receptors are present peripherally on vagal nerve terminals and centrally in the area postrema of the brain. It is not certain whether the action of ondansetron action is mediated peripherally, centrally or both. Cytotoxic drugs and radiation appear to damage gastrointestinal mucosa, causing the release of serotonin from the enterochromaffin cells of the GIT. Stimulation of 5-HT_3 receptors causes transmission of sensory signals to the vomiting centre via vagal afferent fibres to induce vomiting. By binding to 5-HT_3 receptors, ondansetron blocks vomiting mediated by serotonin release.

Ondansetron has no dopamine-receptor antagonist activity.

Name some antiemetics that are safe to use in presence of Parkinsonism.

Ondansetron lacks the adverse effects of dopamine antagonists and is relatively safe to use.

Domperidone is similar to metaclopramide. It acts peripherally. Although it antagonises dopamine, it does not cross the blood brain barrier in significant amounts and hence has negligible extra-pyramidal side effects.

Can you list some side effects of commonly used antiemetics?

- The dopamine antagonist group of drugs carry the potential side effect of causing extra-pyramidal effects.
- Drugs with anticholinergic effects such as hyoscine and cyclizine can cause tachycardia, dry mouth, blurred vision and drowsiness.
- 5-HT_3 receptor antagonists have a favourable side effect profile, but may cause constipation, headache and occasionally derangement of hepatic function.

Q3 Statistical tests

How do you choose an appropriate statistical test?

Choosing the right statistical test depends on the nature of the data, the sample characteristics and the inferences to be made.

Consideration of the nature of data includes:

- Number of variables.
- Type of data (e.g. qualitative, quantitative).

Consideration of the sample characteristics includes:

- Number of groups (e.g. two or more than two).
- Sample type (e.g. normal distribution *parametric* or not *non-parametric*).

What do you mean by P-value?

In statistical terms, P stands for the probability of an event. A 'P-value of 1' always occurs and a 'P-value of 0' never occurs. When testing the difference between samples, the point of interest is in knowing the probability that the difference between the samples is due to chance. It is useful to decide when differences are real rather than due to chance. A probability of 0.05 corresponds to a chance of 1:20.

Conventionally, if the P-value is more than 0.05 it is not statistically significant as there is no difference between the samples (i.e. the differences are not real but are due to chance).

On the other hand if P is less than 0.05 there is a statistically significant difference between the samples (i.e. the differences are real and are not due to chance).

What are α and β errors?

These are also called Type 1 and Type 2 errors.

Type 1 (α) error is 'False positive' where you *assume a difference when there is actually none.*

Type 2 (β) error is 'False negative' where you *assume no difference when there is actually one.*

α error is a statistically accepted error. There is 1:20 chance of making an error of assuming a difference when there is none ($P = 0.05$).

β error is due to small sample size or a large variation in the study population or in situations where even smaller differences are clinically important. In these circumstances, even if a P-value is more than 0.05 it may be statistically insignificant but still clinically relevant. This error can be minimised by increasing the power of study (i.e. increasing the sample size).

What test will you use to analyse qualitative data?
Chi-square test (χ^2).

Can you outline a scheme for choosing the correct statistical test for a given data?

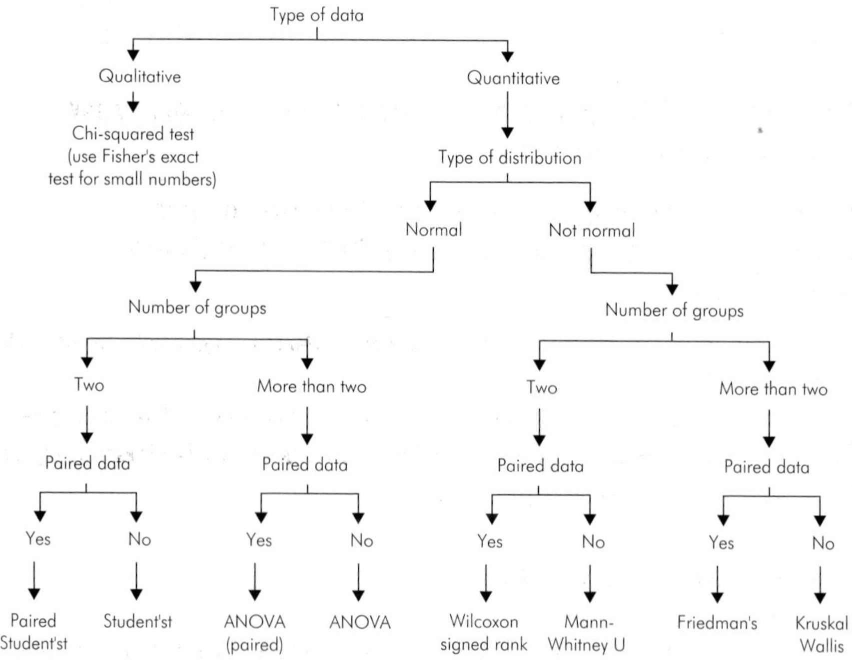

Figure 7.2 *A simple scheme for choosing the correct statistical test*

What is ANOVA?
ANOVA stands for analysis of variance. When testing quantitative data it is used to compare more than two groups then ANOVA is used. The data can be paired or unpaired. In statistics data are considered paired if the two variables to be compared for analysis are from the same patient. With a t-test, as the number of groups

grows, the number of necessary paired comparisons grows quickly. Making multiple comparisons increases the likelihood of finding something by chance – making a Type-1 error. ANOVA puts all the data into one number (F) and gives us *one* P for the null hypothesis.

The mathematics involved with ANOVA is complex but computer software can handle the data.

One potential drawback to an ANOVA is that specificity is lost. The F-value can indicate that there is a significant difference between groups, but not which groups are significantly different from each other. To test for this, a post hoc comparison can be applied to find out where the differences are – which groups are significantly different from each other and which are not.

Clinical 7

Key topics: elderly, ischaemic heart disease, day case, ST depression, consent

Q1 A 70-year-old male is booked for day case unilateral inguinal herniorrhaphy. He has a past history of ischaemic heart disease.

How are elderly patients different from healthy adults with regards to anaesthetic management?

Elderly patients are different from healthy adults physically and physiologically. Morbidity and mortality are higher in elderly patients due to diminished physiological reserves and coexisting pathologies.

Can you list some age-related changes?

- *Respiratory system*:
  - *Physiology*: Over the age of 65 years the closing capacity increases, nearing functional residual capacity even in the sitting position. These patients are more prone to airway collapse, increasing ventilation perfusion mismatch and a resultant increase in the alveolar–arterial oxygen difference. The response to hypoxia and hypercarbia is blunted.
  - *Pathology*: Chest infections, atelectasis.
- *Cardiovascular system*:
  - *Physiology*: Reduced ventricular compliance and myocardial contractility. Vascular compliance is reduced predisposing to swings in blood pressure.

  - *Pathology*: Atherosclerosis, ischaemic heart disease, hypertension and deep vein thrombosis.
- *Nervous system*:
  - *Physiology*: Decreasing density of neurons; reduction in neurotransmitter levels.
  - *Pathology*: Dementia, confusion and risk of cerebrovascular accidents.
- *GIT*:
  - *Physiology*: Reduced competency of lower oesophageal sphincter.
  - *Pathology*: Hiatus hernia.
- *Endocrine and metabolism*:
  - *Physiology*: Lower metabolic rate. Decrease in hormone secretion and responsiveness to hormones, diminishing GFR. Both fluid overload and dehydration are common. Hypothyroidism and diabetes mellitus are more likely. Hypothermia during the peri-operative period is common.
- *Musculoskeletal*:
  - *Physiology*: Calcified ligaments, decreased bone density and poor muscle mass.
  - *Pathology*: Arthritis, pathological fractures and cervical spondylosis.
- *Pharmacology*:
  - Both pharmacokinetics and pharmacodynamics are altered. Multiple polypharmacy carries potential drug interactions.

How will you evaluate a patient with a previous history of ischaemic heart disease?

By history, examination and investigation.

- *History*: History of angina or myocardial infarction, recent angina, palpitations, shortness of breath, syncope, exercise tolerance, drugs, last cardiology consultation, recent change in symptoms, orthopnoea and paroxysmal nocturnal dyspnoea.
- *Examination*: General examination for anaemia, cyanosis, dependent oedema, pulse and blood pressure. Cardiovascular system examination for jugular venous pressure (JVP), Apical impulse, thrill; heart sounds, gallop rhythm, murmurs.
- *Investigation*: As directed by history and examination; electrocardiogram, chest X-ray, echocardiogram, stress ECG, radionucleotide scanning, angiogram.

Why are you concerned about ischaemic heart disease (IHD) in the peri-operative context?

These patients are at a higher risk of peri-operative myocardial infarction. Overall reinfarction rate in these patients is about 6–7%, whereas it is 0.1–0.2% if there is no history of previous myocardial infarction. Peri-operative myocardial infarction has a mortality rate of up to 70%.

What is the significance of the time elapsed from previous myocardial infarction and the risk of peri-operative myocardial infarction?

It is important to establish the timing of previous myocardial infarction. The risk of peri-operative myocardial infarction is high (20–30%) if the time elapsed is less than 3 months, medium (10–20%) if it is 3–6 months and low (4–5%) if it is more than 6 months. The actual level of risk is however uncertain and depends on degree of myocardial insufficiency of individual patients.

What ECG abnormalities are associated with myocardial ischaemia? Why do they happen?

In ischaemia, the myocardial membrane loses its integrity resulting in a leakage of ions. The leakage results in changes in membrane potential and disturbance of current flow. As a result there are ECG changes.

The commonest ECG changes involve the ST segment. It is depressed (>1 mm in limb leads, >2 mm in chest leads) in subendocardial ischemia and elevated in transmural ischaemia.

Ischaemia can also present as conduction abnormalities (heart blocks, bundle branch blocks), arrhythmias (ventricular ectopics, VT, VF), QRS changes (Q waves, poor R wave progression) or T wave changes (isoelectric, inverted).

What are the criteria for doing this procedure as day case?

- *Surgical*: Unilateral inguinal hernia repair is of moderate duration and post-operative pain is mild to moderate and can be managed with simple analgesics and weaker opioids with regional anaesthesia.
- *Medical*: Day surgery is usually restricted to American Society of anaesthesiologists (ASA Grade II). Angina, significant arrhythmia and overt cardiac failure are unacceptable. The 'medical fitness' criteria is controversial and is often locally decided subject to arrangement between the anaesthetist, surgeon and theatre team. Similarly age is not a strict criterion. Geriatric patients are accepted if they are otherwise fit.
- *Social*: Should have appropriate care at home. Carers should be able to understand the post-operative complications. Carers should have an easy access to telephone and transport. They should be living within a reasonable distance so that they are able to get back to the hospital if necessary (within 30 min of travel time).

Assuming the home situation is acceptable, how will you assess the suitability for discharge?

The following are usually required (mnemonic 5*S*)

1 *S*table vitals signs
2 *S*oreness controlled (good pain control)

3 *S*ickness absent (no post-operative nausea and vomiting (PONV))
4 *S*urgical complications nil (controlled bleeding, etc.)
5 *S*ocial parameters acceptable (full orientation and responsiveness, ability to walk, drink, urinate).

What options are available to provide anaesthesia for inguinal herniorrhaphy in this elderly man?

The options available are:

- *General anaesthesia*: Airway: laryngeal mask, endotracheal intubation; Ventilation: spontaneous/controlled.
- *Regional anaesthesia*: Inguinal field block, spinal.
- GA + regional combinations.

Many units do not use spinal anaesthesia unless the clinical situation warrants. This is due to delay in attaining the discharge criteria and more chance of post-dural puncture headache due to early ambulation.

Q2 Critical incident: acute ischaemia

You are proceeding with this case under general anaesthesia with a laryngeal mask airway (LMA) and the patient is breathing spontaneously. He has also had an inguinal field block. Intra-operatively you see this ECG trace in the monitor screen.

What is it and what is the significance?

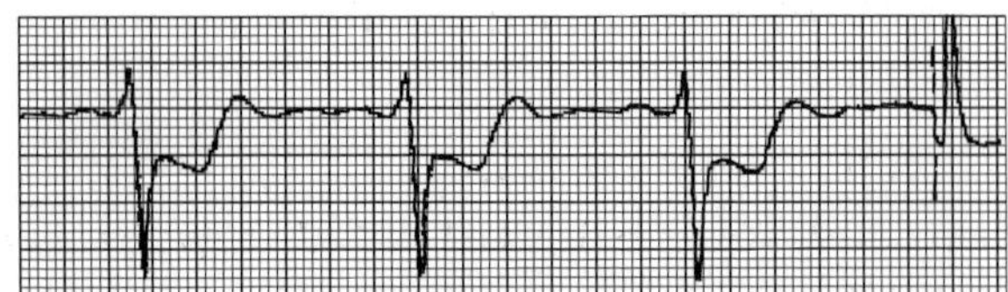

Figure 7.3 *ECG strip: ST depression*

This ECG strip shows ST depression.

ST depression can be due to myocardial ischaemia, hypokalaemia and less commonly due to digoxin therapy. If the depression is more than 1 mm from the isoelectric line in limb leads or more than 2 mm in chest leads it is considered significant. Given the cardiac history, the ST depression in this patient is probably due to myocardial ischaemia.

What will you do now?

- Call for senior help and in the mean time start correcting any obvious insult that might have lead to myocardial ischaemia (bradycardia, tachycardia, hypertension, hypotension, hypoxia, etc.).

- Check the monitors for changes in other parameters, heart rate, SpO_2, $ETCO_2$, blood pressure; check electrode position.
- Tell the surgeon to stop the surgery.

What will be the management strategy for myocardial ischaemia?

Myocardial ischaemia is due to imbalance between the myocardial oxygen supply and demand. The balance is easily tilted in patients with existing heart disease.

Measures to improve myocardial oxygen supply should include administration of 100% oxygen and treatment of hypotension with judicious use of fluids and vasopressors in order to get the required coronary perfusion pressure.

Controlling tachycardia is important as it decreases the diastolic time during which the myocardium is perfused. A blood gas analysis will show impairments in oxygen and carbon dioxide tension. It can also give information about electrolytes and haemoglobin levels. Despite an acceptable haemoglobin level pre-operatively, the haemoglobin level could have dropped due to bleeding and this can precipitate myocardial ischaemia. If so, consider replacement with expanders or blood depending on severity.

To reduce the oxygen demand, optimise the heart rate since tachycardia increases the myocardial oxygen demand. Controlling blood pressure helps in reducing the after load and minimising strain to the ventricles. Drugs like glyceryl trinitrate venodilate and reduce venous return thereby reducing myocardial workload. They also cause coronary vasodilatation and improve perfusion.

How will you manage him post-operatively?

Per-operative myocardial ischaemia detected by ST depression is associated with a high incidence of reinfarction. This patient needs to be admitted in the coronary care unit for intensive monitoring, oxygen supplementation and effective pain relief. Cardiac enzymes need to be tested. Cardiologist input is valuable and subsequent management of this patient depends on the clinical condition and investigation findings.

Q3 Consent

What do you understand by 'consent'?

Consent is a voluntary agreement or approval for a treatment or an investigation. Consent is a person's agreement to allow something to happen after the person has been informed of all the risks involved and the alternatives.

It is not an event but rather a continuous process.

What types of consent are you aware of?

Broadly consent is classified into two types, implied and expressed. Implied consent is assumed from the conduct of the patient. Expressed consent should be oral or writing.

Is there any age limitation to give consent?

In England and Wales, competent young people of any age can give consent for any surgical, medical or dental treatment; it is not necessary to obtain separate consent from the parent or guardian. However, if a person under 18 years of age refuses treatment which is deemed essential, then the patient can be made a ward of Court and the Court may order that an operation may be carried out lawfully. The Court will not order a doctor to perform a procedure.

If a child less than 16 years of age does not want to involve the parents or guardian in consenting what would you do?

If a child under the age of 16 years achieves a sufficient understanding of what is proposed, he or she may consent to treatment. The child must be able to understand the nature, purpose and hazards of the treatment; thus, it is necessary to consider both the age of the child and the nature of the procedure before accepting that the child has sufficient understanding.

The most frequent example in anaesthetic practice involves termination of pregnancy. In these circumstances, if the clinician is satisfied that the child is mature enough to understand the nature of the procedure, common complications and the issues involved and that the requirements of the Abortion Act are met, then he or she may proceed provided that it is considered that to do so without informing the parents is in the child's best interests.

In what situations will you proceed with the treatment without obtaining consent?

- For life-saving procedures when the patient is unconscious or cannot indicate his or her wishes.
- Treatment for physical disorder where the patient is incapable of giving consent by reason of mental incapacity and where the treatment is in the patient's best interests.
- If, during a routine procedure, circumstances suddenly alter and result in a potentially life-threatening situation, a change in the treatment plan may need to be instituted for the benefit of the patient.

If an adult patient is not fit to give consent can another adult consent on his behalf?

No. No other person can consent to treatment on behalf of any adult, including incompetent adults. However, it is prudent to consult with the next of kin before treating an adult without consent.

What do you know about consenting from patients who are Jehovah's Witnesses with respect to blood transfusion?

- If age is less than 16 years and if it is a life-threatening emergency, it is possible to act on the best interest of patient and go ahead with transfusion.
- If age is less than 16 years and it is an elective situation necessitating transfusion then a Court order is required to overrule parents' wishes.
- In an adult, in an elective situation their religious believes are respected and transfusion avoided.

Wishes expressed in the form of an advance directive may need to be considered. The legal situation with regard to these is complex, to say the least. It is also subject to change in line with current moral and political imperatives.

Physics, clinical measurement and safety 7

Key topics: measurement of inhalational anaesthetic agents, pH measurement, breathing systems

Q1 Measurement of inhalational anaesthetic agents

What methods are used to measure the concentration of anaesthetic agent in the fresh gas flow (FGF)?

Gas and vapour analysers can be classified as discrete analysers (extremely accurate) and continuous analysers (less accurate). Discrete analysers are rarely used in clinical anaesthesia. An example of a discrete technique is gas chromatography.

Continuous analysers include:

- Mass spectrometers.
- Raman spectrometers.
- Infrared (IR) analysers.
- Ultraviolet absorption.
- Piezoelectric crystals.
- Refractometer.

What is the principle of gas chromatography?

In this method the unknown gas mixture is injected into a stream of carrier gas (nitrogen, argon or helium) flowing through a column of liquid-coated particles – the stationary phase (e.g. polyethylene glycol). An agent with a low boiling point (volatile) will travel faster through the column. As the gas mixture passes through the column various component gases are slowed down according to their solubility in the stationary phase and thus appear separated out at the end of the column. At the exit end of the column, a detector detects the specific agent and concentration. The detector yields a recording in the form of peaks corresponding to component gases.

This method is very accurate and sensitive but is expensive. It is usually used for research purposes.

How does a mass spectrometer analyse anaesthetic agent?

Mass spectrometers can separate complex mixture of gases. A gas sample is continuously aspirated into a high vacuum chamber where an electron beam ionises the molecules. These molecules become charged ions, and then they are accelerated by an electric field into a final chamber with a magnetic field. Charged ions are deflected by the magnetic field and the radius (arc) of deflection depends on the charge:mass ratio. Lighter ions are deflected most. Detector plates placed at various distances will detect the molecules. The number of detector plates determines the number of gases that can be measured.

Advantages are that it has a rapid response time (<0.1 s) and hence breath-to-breath analysis of a gas sample is possible. The presence of water vapour can interfere with sample measurement and prolong response time. The mass spectrometer is a complex and expensive piece of equipment.

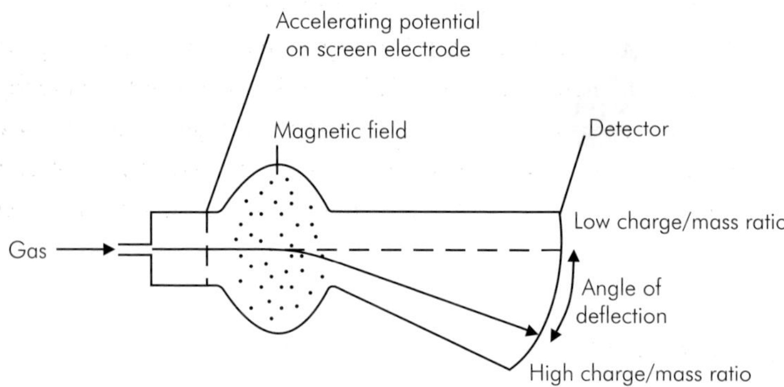

Figure 7.4 *Mass spectrometer*

What is the principle in Raman spectrometry?

In a Raman spectrometer the gas sample is aspirated into the analysing chamber where the molecules interact with monochromatic beam of argon laser. During this stage the rotational energy and vibrational energy of the gas molecules are changed (Raman scattering). Transfer of energy between gas molecules and light results in a change of wavelength which depends on the characteristics of the gas molecule.

What other methods can be used to measure anaesthetic gases and vapours?

- *IR analysers*: Gases having two or more different atoms will absorb IR rays. Different gas molecules absorb specific wavelengths of IR light. By detecting increased absorption at particular frequencies gases can be identified and their concentrations determined.
- *Piezoelectric crystal*: A known voltage is applied to the crystal and this leads to oscillation of the crystal at a particular frequency. There is a thin layer of oil coating over the crystal in which the anaesthetic agent dissolves and it is this that alters the oscillating frequency of the crystal. The change in the resonant frequency is proportional to the dissolved anaesthetic agent. Henry's law states that the quantity of vapour which dissolves is proportional to the partial pressure. Hence partial pressure or concentration of the anaesthetic agent can be measured.
- *UV absorption*: Halogenated vapours will absorb UV light. The only clinical analyser based on this method measures halothane.
- *Refractometer*: When sine waves of the same frequency, amplitude and phase are added, the resulting sine wave will have a greater amplitude. If these two sine waves are 180° out of phase, the resulting sine wave will have zero amplitude and appears as straight line. Addition of sine waves in a variable degree phase difference will result in respective change in the amplitude.

  In a refractometer increased amplitude gives rise to a bright fringe whereas reduced amplitude gives rise to a dark fringe. There are two chambers in the device. One is a reference chamber and the other a sample chamber. The change in the phase of sine waves in the sample chamber and resultant displacement of fringe pattern is dependent on the type and concentration of the anaesthetic agent.

Q2 Measurement of pH

How can you measure the pH of a given blood sample?

pH is measured using an H^+ ion sensitive glass electrode (pH electrode). This is used in most blood gas machines. It consists of two electrodes. One is silver/silver chloride *measuring* electrode and the other one is mercury/mercury chloride *reference* electrode. A potential develops between the two electrodes which depends on the pH difference between the inner buffer solution of the electrode and the blood sample. The H^+ concentration within the pH electrode is maintained constant, so the potential across the electrode is directly proportional to the amount of H^+ ions in the blood sample.

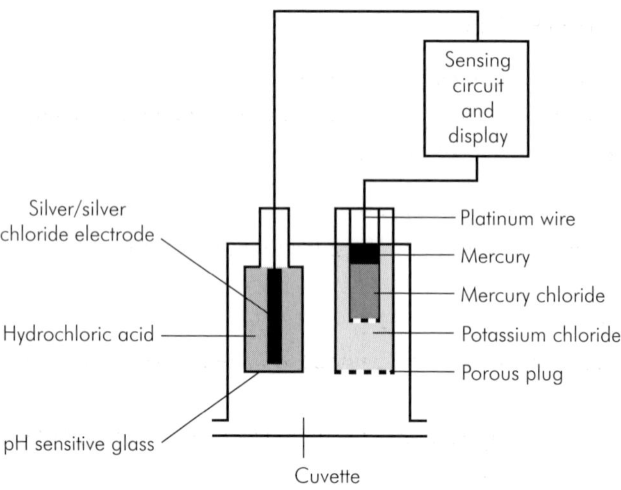

Figure 7.5 *pH electrode*

What factors may give rise to inaccuracy in the reading?

Temperature. Hypothermia increases the solubility of carbon dioxide. Hence $PaCO_2$ is proportionally reduced thereby increasing the pH.

Any holes in the semi-permeable membrane can result in inaccurate reading. Similarly any deposition of protein materials on the electrode will lead to inaccurate values.

How can you calibrate this electrode?

pH electrodes should be regularly calibrated using two buffer solutions of known concentration of H^+ ions.

How do you measure partial pressure of carbon dioxide in a blood sample?

Carbon dioxide combines with water to produce hydrogen ions and hence alters the pH of the electrolyte solution.

$$CO_2 + H_2O \rightarrow H^+ + HCO_3^-$$

The Severinghaus electrode is used to measure partial pressure of carbon dioxide. It consists of a H^+ ion sensitive glass electrode tip of which is covered by nylon mesh and a silver/silver chloride reference electrode. The nylon mesh contains water and bicarbonate. A plastic membrane which is permeable to carbon dioxide separates the blood sample from the electrode.

Q3 Breathing systems

What is the function of a breathing system?

A breathing system delivers oxygen and gases to the patient and helps to eliminate carbon dioxide from the alveolar gas.

How do you classify breathing systems?

Breathing systems can be broadly classified into two groups:

- Open system.
- Closed system.

Closed systems can further be classified into rebreathing and non-rebreathing systems.

Most practical breathing systems behave as semi-closed and partially rebreathing systems.

What do you understand by the term 'rebreathing'?

Rebreathing is inhalation of previously expired gases containing carbon dioxide.

What factors determine rebreathing?

The amount of rebreathing that occurs with any particular anaesthetic breathing system depends on following factors:

- The design of the breathing system.
- The mode of ventilation (spontaneous or controlled).
- The FGF rate.
- Patient's respiratory pattern.

What are the features of an ideal breathing system?

- It should be easy to use and reliable.
- It should have low dead space. Apparatus dead space is the volume between the patient and the expiratory valve. Functional dead space is different from the apparatus dead space which is dependent on the efficiency of the system. It may be greater than the apparatus dead space in an inefficient circuit or less than the apparatus dead space where the FGF flushes out expired gases before inspiration.
- It should not impose any additional inspiratory or expiratory resistance.
- It should protect the patient from barotrauma.
- It should be efficient both for spontaneous and controlled ventilation. It should prevent rebreathing at low FGF.
- It should be economical in using FGF and volatile agents.
- It should permit spontaneous, manual and controlled ventilation in all age groups.

What is a Mapleson A system? Can you draw it?

Mapleson classified breathing systems according to the configuration of the following components:

- Reservoir bag.
- Flexible hosing.
- Adjustable pressure limiting (APL) valve.
- Face mask.

In the Mapleson A system the APL valve is located close to the mask and the reservoir bag is situated near the machine end. A corrugated tube with minimum length of 110 cm (with an internal tidal volume of 550 ml) connects the machine end to the mask. This system was designed by Sir Ivan Magill and hence known as Magill system.

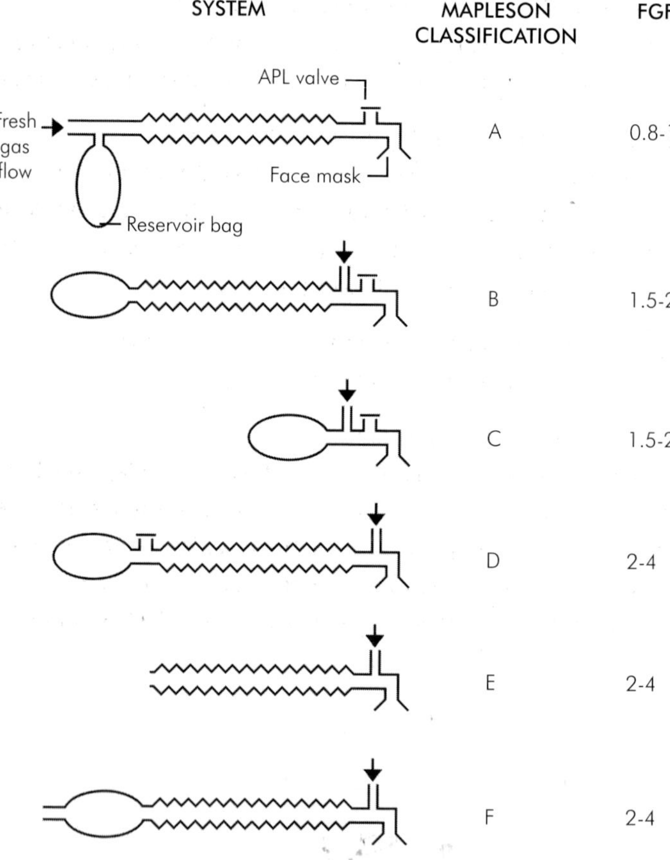

Figure 7.6 *Mapleson classification for breathing systems*

Can you explain the function of Mapleson A system during spontaneous breathing?

During first inspiration whole system is full of fresh gas. During inspiration gases are breathed in from the corrugated tube and reservoir bag.

During early part of expiration expired gas comes from the anatomical dead space (the composition of which is same as fresh gas) and it passes into the corrugated tube towards reservoir bag. During later part of the expiration as the reservoir bag becomes full, the APL valve is opened and alveolar gas is expelled.

During the end expiratory pause the fresh gas continues to flow and washes out the part of alveolar gas which has entered the corrugated tubing.

During next inspiration a mixture of anatomical dead space gas and fresh gas is inhaled.

What is the FGF requirement for spontaneous breathing?

In theory a FGF equal to alveolar ventilation (66% of the minute volume) should be adequate. In practice FGF rate equal to 70–90% of minute volume is necessary.

Can you describe the Bain breathing system?

It is a co-axial Mapleson D system. FGF is delivered through the inner tubing. Expiratory gases are carried through the outer tubing. The APL valve is located close to the reservoir bag. It is less efficient for spontaneous ventilation than Magill system but it is more efficient for controlled ventilation.

What happens if the inner tube is disconnected at the machine end?

It creates a large dead space and leads to rebreathing.

What is an APL valve? How does it work?

It is an adjustable pressure limiting (APL) valve. It contains a lightweight disc which rests on a knife edge seating. The disc is held onto its seating by a spring. The spring is used to adjust the pressure required to open the valve. During spontaneous ventilation valve is in the open position and a pressure of less than 1 cmH_2O is needed to open the valve. During controlled ventilation valve is adjusted to produce a controlled leak.

Physiology 8

Key topics: blood gases, cerebrospinal fluid, metabolism, glucose

Q1 Blood gases

Can you draw the oxygen–haemoglobin dissociation curve?

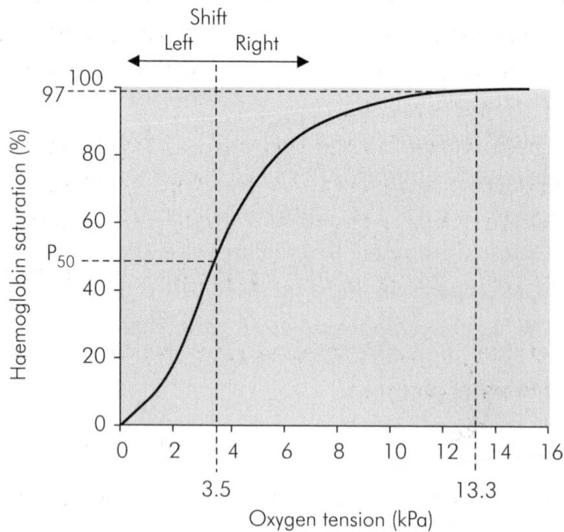

Figure 8.1 *Oxyhaemoglobin dissociation curve*

This is a curve relating the percentage saturation of haemoglobin (y-axis) to the partial pressure of oxygen (x-axis) in blood. The important points on the curve include the venous point at 5.3 kPa (40 mmHg), arterial point at 13.3 kPa (95 mmHg) and P_{50} at 3.56 kPa (26.7 mmHg).

What do you mean by P_{50}?

P_{50} is the partial pressure of oxygen at which haemoglobin is 50% saturated. The position of the curve is best described by the P_{50}. A higher P_{50} implies rightward shift with better oxygen delivery and lower P_{50} implies leftward shift with better oxygen uptake.

Why does it have a sigmoid shape?

The sigmoid shape of the curve is due to the T–R interconversion. In deoxyhaemoglobin the globin units are tightly bound in a tense (T) configuration which reduces the affinity for oxygen. When oxygen is first bound, the bonds holding the globin units are released, producing relaxed configuration (R). This exposes more oxygen binding sites. The combination of first haem in the haemoglobin with oxygen therefore increases the affinity of the second haem for oxygen and so on. This property is described as positive co-operativity.

What do you mean by shifting to the right and left? What factors determine this?

The terms right and left relate to the position of the oxygen dissociation curve and hence the relationship between percentage of saturated haemoglobin and partial pressure of oxygen.

A 'left shift' of the oxygen dissociation curve means an increase in the affinity of haemoglobin for oxygen. Alkalosis, decreased partial pressure of CO_2 (PCO_2), decreased 2,3-diphosphoglycerate (2,3-DPG), decreased temperature and the presence of abnormal haemoglobins such as fetal haemoglobin (HbF) and carboxyhaemoglobin shift the curve to left.

A 'right shift' represents a decrease in affinity of haemoglobin for oxygen. There is therefore enhanced delivery of oxygen to the tissues. Acidosis, increased PCO_2, increased 2,3-DPG and increased temperature shift the curve to right.

How is 2,3-DPG formed? Can you explain the reaction between 2,3-DPG and haemoglobin?

2,3-DPG is formed from 3-phosphoglyceraldehyde which is product of glycolysis via the Embden–Meyerhof pathway.

$$\text{Hb O}_2 + \text{2,3-DPG} \leftrightarrow \text{Hb-2,3-DPG} + \text{O}_2$$

An increase in the concentration of 2,3-DPG shifts the reaction to right causing more oxygen to be released.

What factors affect the concentration of 2,3-DPG?

- Acidosis by inhibiting glycolysis reduces the concentration of 2,3-DPG.
- Thyroid hormone.

- Growth hormone.
- Androgens.
- High altitude.

What is the Bohr effect?

The effect of carbon dioxide on the oxygen dissociation curve is termed the Bohr effect. At tissue level, where PCO_2 is high, carbon dioxide enters the red cells, combines with water to form carbonic acid then dissociating into H^+ and HCO_3^-. The H^+ load shifts the oxygen dissociation curve to the right facilitating the release of oxygen to the tissues.

Can you tell me about carbon dioxide transport?

Carbon dioxide is transported in three forms in blood. Of the 4 ml of carbon dioxide added to each 100 ml of blood from tissues:

- 2.8 ml is carried as bicarbonate (70%).
- 0.9 ml as carbamino compounds (22%).
- 0.3 ml carried in solution (8%).

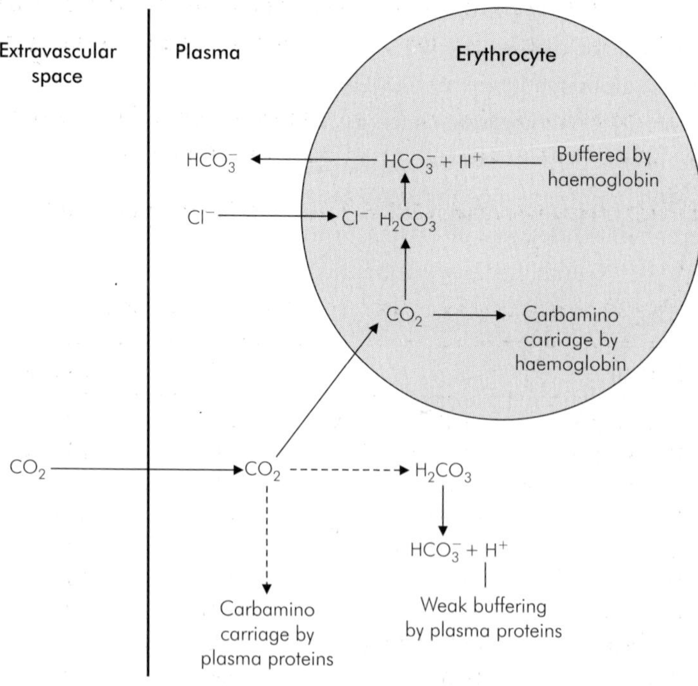

Figure 8.2 *CO_2 transport in blood*

What is the 'chloride shift'?

70% of the carbon dioxide added to the blood from the tissues enters the erythrocyte to form carbonic acid. This is catalysed by carbonic anhydrase. The H_2CO_3 dissociates to give H^+ and HCO_3^-. The HCO_3^- formed diffuses out of the erythrocytes. In order to maintain the electrical neutrality Cl^- enters the red cells. This is called chloride shift.

What do you understand by the Haldane effect?

The influence of the oxygenation state of haemoglobin on the carbon dioxide carrying capacity is described as the Haldane effect. Deoxygenation of haemoglobin enhances carriage of carbon dioxide. This occurs by the activation of H^+ acceptor sites and carbamino formation sites. Oxygenation of haemoglobin causes the reverse effect (as in the lungs) facilitating the 'unloading' of carbon dioxide.

Q2 Cerebrospinal fluid

Describe the formation and circulation of cerebrospinal fluid.

Cerebrospinal fluid (CSF) is formed from the choroid plexus in the lateral ventricles and partly from third and fourth ventricles. From the lateral ventricles circulation reaches the third ventricle through the foramen of Munro. The passage of CSF from third to fourth ventricle happens occurs through the aqueduct foramen. Ultimately CSF leaves the fourth ventricle via the foramina of Magendie (in the **M**idline) and Luschka (**L**aterally) thence reaching the cisterns and bathing the spinal cord and the brain.

CSF is formed at a rate of about 0.3 ml/min (500–600 ml/day). Total volume is 100–150 ml. 85–90% of CSF is reabsorbed through arachnoid villi.

Tell me about the composition of CSF. How does it differ from plasma?

Table 8.1 *Concentrations of major substances in CSF and plasma*

Substance		CSF	Plasma
Protein (g/l)	(g/l)	0.3	70
HCO_3^- (mmol/l)	(mmol/l)	23	25
Glucose	(mmol/l)	4.8	8
Na^+	(mmol/l)	147	150
K^+	(mmol/l)	2.9	4.6
Cl^-	(mmol/l)	112	100
pH	(mmol/l)	7.32	7.4
Osmolality	($mOsm/kgH_2O$)	290	290
PCO_2	(kPa)	6.6	5.3

What are the functions of CSF?

- Protection of brain by providing buoyancy.
- Central chemoreceptor respiratory control.
- Tight control of a chemical environment around the brain.

Describe the role of CSF in respiratory control.

The central chemoreceptors which are sensitive to carbon dioxide are situated in the floor of fourth ventricle and ventral surface of medulla. Carbon dioxide freely diffuses into the CSF. Owing to poor protein content in CSF the buffering mechanism is very limited. Changes in PCO_2 therefore cause more sensitive pH changes in CSF than in plasma. An increase in PCO_2 therefore stimulates the respiratory centre to produce hyperventilation by acting on the central chemoreceptors. If this is sustained, a slow compensatory mechanism comes into play. This is due to secretion of bicarbonate into CSF, buffering the pH.

Q3 Metabolism

Define metabolic rate. What is basal metabolic rate?

Metabolic rate is energy liberated per unit time. Basal metabolic rate (BMR) is the metabolic rate of a subject under standardised conditions at mental and physical rest, in a comfortable environmental temperature and fasted for 12 h.

What is the normal BMR?

In a healthy adult it is about 70–100 kcal/h.

How do you measure the BMR?

BMR can be estimated by direct and indirect methods.

The direct method uses a whole body calorimeter. Water flows steadily through the calorimeter and the temperature rise of the water is measured after placing the subject within the calorimeter chamber. This temperature change is proportional to the heat produced per hour.

The indirect method employs the measurement of oxygen consumption using an oxygen-filled spirometer and a carbon dioxide absorbing system. The amount of oxygen consumption (ml) is corrected for temperature and pressure.

The energy production = 4.82 kcal/l of oxygen consumed.
Example: 250 ml/min oxygen consumption, i.e. 0.25 l/min
$0.25 \times 60 \times 24 = 360$ l/day.
Therefore, energy produced = $360 \times 4.82 = 1735$ kcal.

Can you name some factors affecting metabolic rate?

Height, weight, surface area, age, sex, exercise, temperature, emotional state, recent ingestion of food, hormones (thyroxine, epinephrine), pregnancy, menstruation and some disease conditions such as sepsis.

What is the normal plasma glucose level?

3.9–6.1 mmol/l.

What is glycolysis?

Glycolysis is the breakdown of glucose to pyruvate or lactate. The pathway is called the Embden–Meyerhof pathway and this takes place in the cytoplasm of cells. Glycolysis can happen both in aerobic and anaerobic environments. In anaerobic glycolysis the net energy gain is only two ATP molecules and there is an accumulation of lactate.

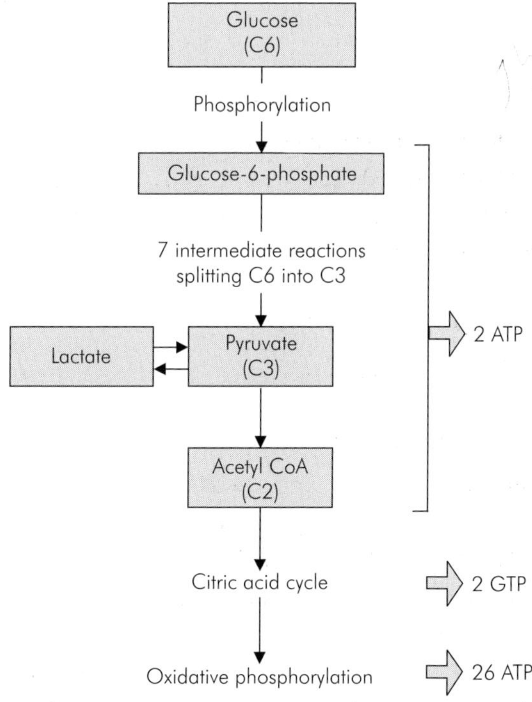

Figure 8.3 *Glycolysis*

Can you describe the phosphorylation of glucose? Where does it occur and what are the enzymes involved?

Glucose is phosphorylated to form glucose-6-phosphate. This reaction is catalysed by *hexokinase* in tissue cells and *glucokinase* (*glucose-6-phosphatase*) in liver cells.

Liver glucokinase has greater specificity for glucose and is increased by insulin and decreased by diabetes and starvation.

Further glucose catabolism proceeds via two different routes:

- Cleavage through fructose to trioses (Embden–Meyerhof pathway) [fructose-6-phosphate, fructose 1,6-diphosphate to pyruvate].
- Through 6-phosphogluconate and the pentoses to phosphoglyceraldehyde (direct oxidative pathway, hexose monophosphate shunt).

What happens to glucose-6-phosphate?

Glucose-6-phosphate is either polymerised into glycogen or catabolised via glycolytic pathway.

What is gluconeogenesis?

Gluconeogenesis is the conversion of non-glucose molecules into glucose. Examples are glycerol, amino acids, pyruvate and lactate.

What is the citric acid cycle?

The citric acid cycle and oxidative phosphorylation are the common end pathways for the products of carbohydrate, lipid and protein metabolism. They take place in mitochondria and are the final events of the energy producing machinery in metabolism. Acetyl-CoA (C2) enters the citric acid cycle. It combines with oxaloacetate (C4) to form citrate (C6). This passes around a cycle and results in energy production in the form of six NADH, two $FADH_2$ and two GTP per molecule of glucose.

The NADH and $FADH_2$ enter the oxidative phosphorylation process to generate ATP.

Pharmacology 8

Key topics: NSAIDs, anti-arrhythmics and isomerism

Q1 NSAIDs

Can you name some non-steroidal anti-inflammatory drugs?

The NSAIDs are heterogeneous class of drugs grouped together by their common anti-inflammatory, analgesic and anti-pyretic properties. They can be classified based on their chemical structure.

- *Enolic acids*: Piroxicam, meloxicam, tenoxicam and phenylbutazone.
- *Acetic acid derivatives*: Diclofenac, ketorolac and indomethacin.
- *Salicylic acid derivatives*: Aspirin.
- *Propionic acid derivatives*: Ibuprofen and ketoprofen.

They can also be classified based on their mechanism of action.

- *Non-specific cyclo-oxygenase (COX) inhibitors*: Aspirin, diclofenac, ibuprofen.
- *Preferential COX-2 inhibitors*: Meloxicam.
- *Specific COX-2 inhibitors*: Celecoxib, parecoxib and rofecoxib.

These drugs are used to treat mild to moderate postoperative pain and treatment of chronic inflammatory conditions.

What is the mechanism of their action?

In spite of their structural variation all NSAIDs share a common mechanism of action.

They produce their action by interfering with the production of prostaglandins. They inhibit the enzyme COX thereby preventing the production of both prostaglandins and thromboxanes from membrane phospholipids. Aspirin produces irreversible inhibition of the enzyme whereas other NSAIDs produce reversible inhibition.

How are prostaglandins formed and what are the effects of various prostaglandins?

Arachidonic acid is a major component of cell membrane phospholipids and the enzyme COX converts arachidonic acid to cyclic endoperoxides. The spectrum of prostaglandins formed depends on the property of the tissue. In most of the tissues, cyclic endoperoxides are converted to prostaglandin E_2, F_2 and D_2 in response to tissue injury. In platelets the cyclic endoperoxides are converted into thromboxane-A_2 (TXA_2), which induces platelet aggregation adhesion and vasoconstriction. In vascular endothelial cells prostacyclin is produced which inhibits platelet aggregation and causes vasodilatation.

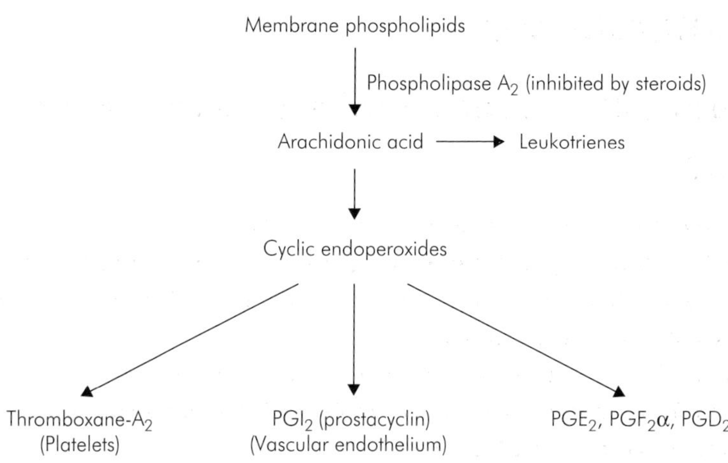

Figure 8.4 *Formation of prostaglandins*

Can you tell me more about COX enzymes?

There are two isoforms of COX enzyme, COX-1 and COX-2. COX-1 (the constitutive form) is responsible for production of TXA_2 in the platelets, PGE_2 in the kidneys and prostacyclin in the endothelial cells and gastric mucosa.

COX-2 (inducible form) is induced when tissues are exposed to inflammatory stimuli. It is produced in macrophages, endothelial cells and synovial cells following trauma to the tissues.

Under normal conditions COX-1 activity predominates and adverse effects are produced by inhibition of prostaglandins normally associated with homeostatic control and control of blood flow. COX-2 is responsible for most of the prostaglandins produced during inflammation and the clinical effect of analgesia is mediated by inhibition of the induced COX-2 isoform.

What do you know about the pharmacokinetics of diclofenac?

Diclofenac is well absorbed in the acid environment of stomach, it has high hepatic metabolism and hence bioavailability is 60%. In general other NSAIDs have low first pass metabolism. It is highly protein bound (99.5%) and therefore has potential for displacing other drugs from plasma proteins. It can therefore potentiate the effects of oral anti-coagulants, anti-convulsants, lithium and oral hypoglycaemic agents. It has a small volume of distribution. It is metabolised in the liver by hydroxylation and conjugation into inactive metabolites. The metabolites are partly excreted in the urine (60%) and bile (40%).

What is the benefit of using NSAIDs along with opioids for postoperative analgesia?

NSAIDs provide analgesia for moderate to severe pain. When used in combination with opioids they have been shown to have variable opioid sparing effect up to 60%. This may result in improved analgesia and reduction in opioid-related side effects. There is no tolerance to NSAIDs.

What are the adverse effects of NSAIDs?

- *Gastrointestinal system*: NSAIDs cause dyspepsia, nausea, bleeding from gastric or duodenal vessels and mucosal ulceration. Prostaglandins play an important role in maintaining gastric mucosal blood flow and in reducing gastric acid secretion. Selective COX-2 inhibitors are associated with a reduced incidence of gastrointestinal complications.
- *Respiratory*: Some of the prostaglandins cause bronchodilatation and hence blocking prostaglandin secretion may lead to bronchospasm in susceptible individuals. Acute severe asthma may be precipitated in 10–20% of asthmatics when

given NSAIDs. By inhibiting prostaglandin production, more of the arachidonic acid is converted to leukotrienes which can cause bronchospasm.

- *Renal*: NSAIDs impair renal function and may cause acute renal failure. Renal prostaglandins are important in maintenance of renal blood flow and glomerular filtration when blood flow is borderline. NSAIDs may precipitate fluid retention and this may be significant in patients with cardiac failure.

Are there any risk factors that may precipitate impaired renal function?

Risk factors for impaired renal function include elderly patients, co-administration of angiotensin-converting enzyme inhibitors (ACEI), diuretics, cardiac failure, hypotension and hypo-volaemia.

- *Haematological*: Inhibition of COX disturbs the balance of prostacyclin and TXA_2. There is reduced production of TXA_2 which reduces platelet aggregation and also prevents vasoconstriction. As aspirin produces irreversible enzyme inhibition, the effect on platelet function lasts for the life span (7–10 days) of platelets. Other NSAIDs may have a reversible effect on the enzyme, hence the platelet function can return to normal once the drug is eliminated from the body.

  Hepatic damage is normally observed following prolonged and excessive use of NSAIDs.
- *Drug interactions*: As NSAIDs are highly protein bound, they can displace anticoagulants such as heparin and warfarin from their protein binding sites and increase their effect.

Can you name some NSAIDs which are specific COX-2 inhibitors?

Celecoxib and parecoxib are specific COX-2 inhibitors. They significantly reduce the gastrointestinal complications and they do not affect the platelet function. There is growing awareness about increased incidence of thrombo-embolic events in susceptible patients taking COX-2 inhibitors. Rofecoxib has been withdrawn from clinical use. Research implying increased risks of myocardial infarction (MI) and cerebrovascular accident (CVA) in chronic usage is emerging.

Q2 Anti-arrhythmics

Can you name some drugs that can be used to treat atrial fibrillation?

Digoxin, amiodarone and bisoprolol can be used to control the heart rate in atrial fibrillation.

How do you classify anti-arrhythmic drugs?

Anti-arrhythmic drugs can be classified into four classes (Vaughan Williams, 1970) based on their effect on the cardiac action potential.

- Class I drugs produce Na^+ channel blockade. Blockade of Na^+ channel results in reduced rate and amplitude of phase 0 depolarisation. They are further classified according to their effect on the refractory period of cardiac muscle.
  - Class Ia drugs prolong the refractory period (QT interval is prolonged).
  - Class Ib drugs reduce the duration of refractory period (QT interval is reduced).
  - Class Ic drugs have no effect on refractory period (no effect on QT interval).
- Class II drugs include β blockers, which competitively block the effect of catecholamines. They prolong the duration of phase 4 (increase the refractory period) and decrease automaticity.
- Class III drugs produce K^+ channel blockade and prolong repolarisation, hence they increase the duration of effective refractory period.
- Class IV include calcium channel blockers [verapamil and diltiazem (nifedipine does not have anti-arrhythmic effect)]. They slow the action potential upstroke in the sinoatrial (SA) and atrioventricular (AV) nodes, and prolong the plateau of phase 2 in atrial and ventricular tissue.

Table 8.2 *Vaughan Williams classification*

Drug	Action	Examples
Class Ia	Na^+ channel blockers; prolongs the refractory period	Quinidine, procainamide, disopyramide
Class Ib	Na^+ channel blockers; shortens the refractory period	Lidocaine, mexiletine, phenytoin
Class Ic	Na^+ channel blockers; no significant effect refractory period	Flecainide, encainide
Class II	Beta-adrenergic blockers	Propranolol, timolol, atenolol
Class III	Potassium channel blockers that prolong repolarisation	Amiodarone, sotalol
Class IV	Slow calcium channel blockers	Verapamil, diltiazem

In addition to above classes there are also other drugs such as digoxin, adenosine, magnesium which can be grouped as miscellaneous.

Can you explain how amiodarone acts as an anti-arrhythmic?

Amiodarone is a class III anti-arrhythmic drug. It also has weak class I, class II and class IV action. It blocks the K^+ channels and slows the rate of repolarisation thereby increasing the duration of the action potential. It also prolongs the effective refractory period.

Can you describe the pharmacokinetics of amiodarone?

Amiodarone is poorly absorbed from the gut with a bioavailability of 50% to 70%. It is about 95% protein bound. It has a very long half-life which varies from 20 to 100 days. It has a large apparent volume of distribution (70 l/kg). A considerable amount of the drug is stored in fat and other tissues. Its metabolite desmethylamiodarone has some anti-arrhythmic activity. It is excreted by lacrimal glands, skin and biliary tract.

What are the clinical uses of amiodarone?

It is used in the treatment of most tachyarrhythmias. It is particularly useful for the treatment of supraventricular tachycardia (SVT), ventricular tachycardia (VT) and Wolff–Parkinson–White (WPW) syndrome. A loading dose of 5 mg/kg over an hour followed by 15 mg/kg over 24 h is used for intravenous use. It can also be used orally as 200 mg thrice daily for the first week and then slowly reduced to 200 mg once daily.

What are the side effects of amiodarone?

Side effects are common with amiodarone (more than 75% of patients receiving drug) and the incidence increases after a year of treatment.

- Pulmonary toxicity and fibrosis (10–15%, can cause death in 10% of those affected). This can be reversed if the treatment is stopped early enough.
- Hepatic dysfunction (cirrhosis, hepatitis and jaundice), this can be irreversible. Liver function tests should be performed regularly.
- Asymptomatic corneal deposits occur in most patients.
- Central nervous system effects (ataxia, dizziness, depression, nightmares, hallucinations).
- Hypothyroidism or hyperthyroidism has been observed. Amiodarone prevents peripheral conversion of T_4 to T_3.
- Cutaneous photosensitivity (25% of patients) and blue-grey discolouration of skin (less than 5% of patients).
- Peripheral neuropathy.

What are the clinical uses of digoxin?

Digoxin is used in the treatment of atrial fibrillation and flutter. It is also used in the treatment of cardiac failure.

What is the mechanism of action of digoxin?

It inhibits Na^+, K^+ ATPase enzyme, leading to increased intracellular Na^+, and decreased intracellular K^+ concentration. As a result of increased intracellular Na^+ there is increased influx of Ca^{2+} into the cell in exchange to Na^+. Increased intracellular Ca^{2+} increases excitability and force of myocardial contractility.

Digoxin increases the refractory period of the AV node and bundle of His but decreases the ventricular refractory period. Digoxin also acts indirectly by enhancing the release of acetylcholine at the cardiac muscarinic receptors. This effect is antagonised by atropine.

Tell me how digoxin is cleared from the body.

It is mainly excreted in the unchanged form in kidneys, only a small proportion is metabolised in the liver.

What are the side effects of digoxin?

Side effects of digoxin are usually dose dependent and occur at dosages higher than those needed to achieve a therapeutic effect.

- Cardiovascular side effects include various arrhythmias and conduction disturbances. Electrocardiographical (ECG) changes such as prolonged PR-interval, ST-segment depression and short QT-interval may be seen.
- Gastrointestinal effects include nausea, vomiting, diarrhoea.
- Headache and visual disturbances are common side effects.

How will you recognise digoxin toxicity?

Digoxin has a low therapeutic ratio; hence toxicity is more likely when the plasma concentration exceeds the therapeutic level. A plasma concentration of more than 2.5 μg/l is associated with toxic effects. Whenever possible, plasma levels of digoxin should be monitored to avoid toxicity.

Initial effects are related gastrointestinal upset (i.e. anorexia, nausea, vomiting and abdominal discomfort). Neurological effects include fatigue, headache and visual disturbances are frequently seen.

The commonest arrhythmias include ventricular extra systoles, VT and various types of AV block. Hypokalaemia, hypomagnesaemia and hypocalcaemia can exacerbate cardiac toxicity.

How can you treat digoxin toxicity?

- Hypokalaemia should be corrected.
- Ventricular arrhythmias may be treated with phenytoin and lidocaine.
- Digoxin-specific antibody fragments (Fab) can be used to treat severe arrhythmias. Fab binds to digoxin and forms digoxin–fab complex which is removed from the circulation by kidneys.

Q3 Isomerism

What are isomers?

Isomers are defined as compounds that have the same molecular formula, but different structures. They have the same molecular weight and the same chemical composition but different structural arrangement.

What are the types of isomers?

There are two main types, structural isomers and stereoisomers.

1 *Structural isomers* have the same molecular formula but different connections (bonding) between the atoms. Hence they have different chemical structures.
2 *Stereoisomers* have the same molecular formula, same connections between the atoms, but different arrangements of atoms in three-dimensional space.

Can you give some examples for structural isomers?

They can be further classified into three groups:

1 *Chain isomerism*: Carbon skeleton varies with the isomers whilst retaining same functional group (e.g. butane and isobutene).
2 *Position isomerism*: Carbon skeleton is identical but the component atoms or functional groups are in different positions (e.g. enflurane and isoflurane).
3 *Dynamic isomerism (tautomerism)*: A given molecule exists in two forms. Change from one form to another is precipitated by change in physical environment, such as a change in pH. For example, midazolam is ionised at acidic pH but changes structure by forming an unionised ring when injected into blood at physiological pH of 7.4.

Can you give some examples for stereoisomers?

There are two types of stereoisomers, geometric isomers and enantiomers.

1 *Geometric isomers*: These have the same covalent bond (attached by a carbon atom) but a difference in the spatial arrangement of atoms. If the groups of atoms are on the same side of the covalent bond or ring, then the arrangement is called *cis* and if the groups are on opposite side of plane of the covalent bond, it is called *trans*.

   Mivacurium contains three geometric isomers, *trans–trans, cis–cis* and *cis–trans*. Atracurium has 10 stereoisomers, cisatracurium is but one of them.
2 *Enantiomers*: These are molecules that appear to be mirror images of each other. They have a middle asymmetric carbon atom which is attached to four different groups of atoms.

What do you understand by the term chirality?

Any compound that has a mirror image that is different from itself is chiral (Greek word cheir means hand). A chiral centre is a carbon atom or quaternary nitrogen surrounded by four different chemical groups. Chirality is the property of 'handedness'. If a left hand glove is placed in front of the mirror, it looks like a glove that fits into the right hand and vice versa. Right and left hands are mirror images of each other. These isomers have identical physical and chemical properties. They have the same boiling point, density and colour, they differ only the way they interact with plane-polarised light.

An intravenous infusion must be started preoperatively and undue length of starvation avoided.

Intraoperatively, standard anaesthetic techniques can be used, adhering to the goals. Measures to minimise heat loss and meticulous care to avoid any stagnation of blood (as due to poor positioning) should be taken.

Postoperatively these precautions should continue. Oxygen supplementation is advocated. In severe disease forms with 'painful infarction crises' in the past, post-operative pain control may be challenging and needs to be properly addressed.

The surgeon wants to use a tourniquet for the arthroscopy. Are you happy about that?

In sickle cell trait though some advocate thorough exsanguination of the limb and application of tourniquet to be safe, in general both homozygote and heterozygote form of the disorder are considered to be contraindications for the application of a tourniquet. Intravenous regional anaesthesia is contraindicated. The surgeon should have sufficient skill and experience to proceed without a tourniquet.

Can this case be done in a day case setting?

Possibly. It is determined by the nature of surgery and severity of the disease. Patients with sickle cell trait for minor surgical procedures can be done in day case setting. Sickle cell anaemia is considered a contraindication for most day-case surgery.

Q2 Critical incident: failed intubation

You are anaesthetising a young female for urgent appendicectomy. After performing rapid sequence induction you cannot see the vocal cords during laryngoscopy.

What are the different grades of view at laryngoscopy?

Cormack and Lehane graded laryngoscopic views into:

- *Grade I*: Complete visualisation of vocal cords.
- *Grade II*: Only posterior portion of laryngeal aperture seen.
- *Grade III*: Only epiglottis seen.
- *Grade IV*: Visualisation of soft palate only.

In this patient, what are you going to do?

First take simple measures to improve the grading of the view at laryngoscopy. These include re-positioning the head and neck with appropriate neck flexion and head extension. Using a different blade, a longer or straight one may be helpful. Use of gentle external pressure applied to thyroid cartilage can improve the view. If a Grade I or II view is possible, carry on with intubation with or without the aid of gum elastic bougie.

With all these manoeuvres there is no improvement in the view. What will you do?

After two to three proper attempts this is an unexpected failed intubation. Summon senior help. Primary aims are to:

- Provide oxygenation.
- Protect airway by continuing cricoid pressure.
- Ensure hypnosis till the muscle relaxant effect wears off.

Maintaining cricoid pressure, try bag and mask ventilation with 100% oxygen. Inserting an oropharyngeal airway may be helpful. Having two persons, one to hold the mask and another to squeeze the bag can make the ventilation more effective. Avoid over-vigorous mask ventilation that can distend stomach with gas and increase the chance of regurgitation. If bag and mask ventilation is possible and oxygenation is maintained then allow spontaneous breathing and wake her up. Later, with expert help, a definitive airway can be planned.

What options are available if this becomes a 'cannot intubate cannot ventilate' scenario?

- A laryngeal mask airway (LMA) can be tried. If ventilation is possible then wake the patient up.
- If ventilation is not possible even with a LMA and if the patient continues to desaturate, proceed to an emergency cricothyroid puncture.

The LMA can also be used as a guide to pass a proper endotracheal tube. An intubating LMA (ILMA) is more appropriate in this circumstance. With the help of an experienced anaesthetist fibre-optic intubation can be performed through the LMA or ILMA.

What are the different ways by which you can secure a definitive airway in an anticipated difficult intubation?

- Awake fibre-optic intubation.
- Gas induction and laryngoscopy whilst preserving spontaneous breathing.
- Elective surgical airway under local anaesthesia.

Q3 Preoperative assessment

What is the purpose of a preoperative visit?

The preoperative visit is an important strategy that provides an opportunity to optimise the patient in order to minimise peri-operative morbidity and mortality.

The anaesthetist gets a chance to introduce and explain his role, assess the patient in order to evaluate the functional reserve, identify the coexisting morbidities and correct the reversible factors, allay the anxiety of patient and if needed, premedicate.

Tell me about the ASA scoring system.

American Society of Anesthesiologists (ASA) scoring system relates to the preoperative condition of the patient. With increasing scores the peri-operative mortality increases. See SOE 6.

How do you assess the airway?

By history, examination and investigation.

- *History*: Previous 'difficult airway alerts', surgery or injury to the head and neck, radiotherapy, snoring, obstructive sleep apnoea, neurological disorders.
- *Examination* (Mnemonic: MOUTHS):
  M: Mandible, retrognathia
  O: Opening of mouth, inter-incisor distance
  U: Uvula, Mallampati scoring
  T: Teeth, dentures, missing teeth, loose teeth, crowded teeth
  H: Head, movement in the neck, thyromental distance
  S: Silhouette, Obesity
- *Investigations*: X-ray, nasal-endoscopy, CT-scan.

How do you assess the Mallampatti score? What are the classes?

The patient sits opposite to the anaesthetist with mouth open and tongue protruded. Depending on the structures visualised in the back of the mouth four classes are described:

- *Class 1*: Faucial pillars, soft palate and uvula seen.
- *Class 2*: Faucial pillars and soft palate seen. Base of tongue masks uvula.
- *Class 3*: Only soft palate visible.
- *Class 4*: Even soft palate not visible.

What are the Wilson risk factors?

This is another scoring system to predict difficult intubation. The five risk factors included are:

- Obesity.
- Restricted head and neck movements.
- Restricted jaw movements.
- Receding mandible.
- Buck teeth.

Each factor can score 0–2 points, to give a maximum of 10 points.

Physics, clinical measurement and safety 8

Key topics: cerebral oxygen consumption, pressure gauge, measurement of pressure, pneumotachograph

Q1 Cerebral oxygen consumption

How can you monitor cerebral blood flow?

Cerebral blood flow (CBF) can be monitored using transcranial Doppler ultrasonography (TCD). Using jugular bulb oximetry, arterio-venous oxygen content difference can be determined, and this is proportional to CBF. Other techniques such as nitrous oxide wash-in, xenon computed tomography, single photon emission computed tomography are available but not widely used.

What is the principle of TCD?

The principle of Doppler shift. The difference between the transmitted and reflected ultra-sound frequency is known as Doppler shift, the magnitude of which is related to the velocity of the reflector (red cells in the blood vessel). By integrating velocity with cross-sectional area of the blood vessel, flow rate can be calculated.

Which artery is commonly chosen?

The middle cerebral artery is chosen as it is accessible through temporal window, just above the zygomatic arch.

What is the normal CBF?

Normal CBF is 54 ± 12 ml/100 g/min.

What are the clinical uses of TCD?

TCD is used in following clinical situations:

- During carotid endarterectomy to monitor CBF.
- To detect emboli both for micro-emboli and gas emboli.
- In subarachnoid haemorrhage to detect vasospasm.

How do you monitor cerebral oxygen consumption?

Cerebral oxygen consumption can be monitored using jugular bulb oximetry.

Jugular bulb oxygen saturation ($SjvO_2$) is measured and oxygen content is calculated. Arterial oxygen content is calculated by measuring arterial oxygen saturation. The difference between these two is cerebral oxygen consumption.

What can cause reduced jugular bulb oxygen saturation?

Low values for $SjvO_2$ may be seen in following conditions:

- Reduced arterial oxygen content due to anaemia or hypoxaemia.
- Reduced CBF due to hypotension, vasospasm or intracranial hypertension.
- Increased cerebral oxygen consumption due to increased metabolism due to fever and seizures.

How else you can monitor cerebral oxygenation?

Cerebral oxygenation can be monitored using near-infrared spectroscopy (NIRS).

What is the principle used in NIRS?

Near-infrared light (700–1000 nm) applied to the scalp, penetrates to a depth of several centimetres and then reflected back to scalp. During the path, light is absorbed by haemoglobin, oxyhaemoglobin and myoglobin. The difference between the emitted and reflected light is proportional to the CBF. Micro-catheters incorporating miniature Clark electrode can be directly inserted into the brain parenchyma can be used measure PO_2.

Q2 Pressure regulators

What is the pressure in an oxygen cylinder?

It is 137 bar.

What is the pressure in the oxygen pipe line?

It is 4 bar.

What is the pressure at fresh gas flow outlet in an anaesthetic machine?

It is reduced to less than 2 cmH_2O.

How is this pressure reduced?

Cylinder pressure is reduced to a constant operating pressure of 4 bar using a pressure regulator (pressure reducing valve). The pipeline pressure is reduced to 1–2 bar using a second stage pressure regulator or a flow restrictor. Then, as the gas passes through the flow meters and long tubes, pressure is further reduced to a safe level before exiting through the fresh gas outlet.

Pressure = force/area. As the cross-sectional area of the conducting tubing increases the pressure drops. The pipeline system within the machine is designed in such a way that there is a progressive increase in the size of the conducting tubes from the central supply to the patient end. This design also contributes to the drop in pressure.

How does a pressure regulator work?

It consists of two chambers, a high-pressure chamber (P) and a low-pressure (p) control chamber. These chambers are separated by small conical inlet valve which is coupled to a large diaphragm. A constant force is exerted on the diaphragm by a spring (F), which controls the pressure in the control chamber (supply pressure). As the pressure in the control pressure chamber decreases, the force acting on the diaphragm decreases and the conical valve moves downwards and allows more gas into the chamber. The relationship between the force acting on the diaphragm and conical valve is given by

$$F = Pa + pA,$$

where F = Force exerted by the spring, P = high inlet pressure, p = pressure in the control chamber, a = area of the conical valve and A = area of the diaphragm.

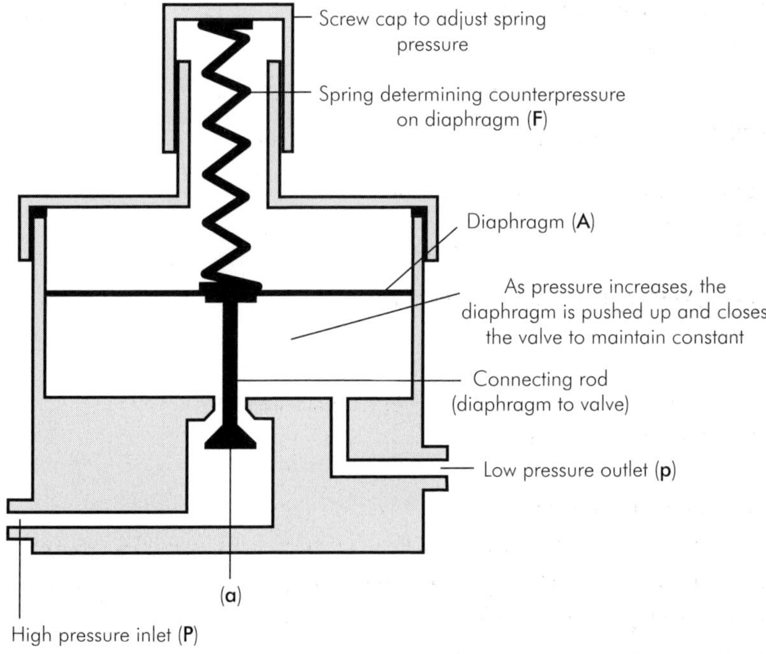

Figure 8.5 *Single-stage pressure regulator*

Q3 Pressure measurement

Can you define pressure?

Pressure is defined as force per unit area.

What units are used to measure pressure?

Depending upon what is measured, a variety of units for pressure is used. The SI unit is the Pascal. When describing blood pressure it is mmHg; partial pressure of gases in kPa; airway pressure in cmH_2O; cylinder pressure in bar or psi.

1 atmosphere (atm) = 760 Torr or;

760 mmHg = 1033 cmH_2O = 101 kPa = 14.7 psi = 1 bar.

How do you measure the pressure in a cylinder?

It is measured using a pressure gauge. A Bourdon pressure gauge is commonly used in anaesthetic machines.

What are the components of this gauge?

It consists of a robust, flexible, coiled tube which has an oval cross-section. One end of the tube is exposed to the inside of cylinder or gas supply and the other end is sealed and connected to a needle pointer which moves over a dial.

How does this gauge work?

The pressure in the cylinder causes the coiled tube to uncoil and this movement moves the needle. The position of the needle corresponds to the pressure inside the cylinder.

What are the advantages?

The Bourdon gauge is simple technology, which is robust and can be used to measure high pressures. It will operate in any position and does not require a power supply.

What are the disadvantages?

It is not suitable for low pressures. It is not easy to calibrate.

What is gauge pressure and what is absolute pressure?

Gauge pressure is pressure above the atmospheric pressure as directly measured by the pressure gauge whereas absolute pressure includes atmospheric pressure.

[absolute pressure = gauge pressure + atmospheric pressure]

Can you name any other pressure gauges?

An aneroid gauge is used to measure low pressures such as blood pressure.

What is the mechanism in an aneroid gauge?

It contains a capsule or a bellow, one end of which is connected to a needle pointer and the other end is exposed to the sampled pressure. When it is connected to the sampled pressure, the bellow expands and moves the pointer over a scale.

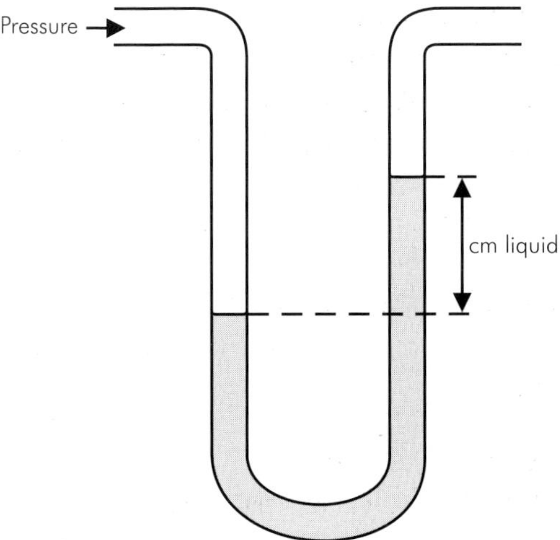

Figure 8.6 *Manometer*

How else the pressure can be measured?

A simple manometer and piezo-resistive strain gauge can be used to measure pressure.

A manometer is a most basic and simple device. It is used for calibrating other devices. It consists of tube filled with liquid. An unknown pressure is measured by balancing it against the pressure due to the column of liquid.

What liquids are commonly used?

Water and mercury are commonly used and hence the pressure is expressed as cmH_2O or mmHg.

What are the advantages of a manometer?

It is a simple device and does not need calibration.

What are the disadvantages of this?

It is bulky and lacks a direct reading. There is a potential for parallax error (this is an error that can occur if the reading is not read in line with the level of the liquid).

What is the principle in the piezo-resistive strain gauge?

It consists of a semiconductor material with piezo-resistive properties. When subjected to mechanical strain, the resistance changes and the change in electrical resistance results in a small current flow which can be amplified and processed. The semiconductor is deposited on a thin diaphragm which is exposed to the sample pressure. The distortion of diaphragm is proportional to the amount of pressure. The distortion of diaphragm produces a strain in the piezo-resistive material that leads to the change in the resistance. This change in resistance results in a small current signal from the transducer.

- *Advantages*: It is versatile and it is suitable for on line display of pressure reading. It can also be adapted for measuring differential pressures.
- *Disadvantages*: It requires a power supply and signal processing unit.

How can you measure tidal volume in a patient who is anaesthetised in theatre?
Wright's respirometer and pnuemotachographs can be used to measure tidal volume.

How does the Wright respirometer work?
It consists of a rotating vane which is attached to a pointer by means of clockwork gear mechanism. It can be used to measure the volume for a unidirectional gas flow. It usually positioned on the expiratory side of the breathing system. The gas flow rotates the vane, the number of revolutions depend on the total volume of gas flow which passes. The revolutions of the vane causes pointer to rotate over the display dial, giving a direct reading of tidal volume.

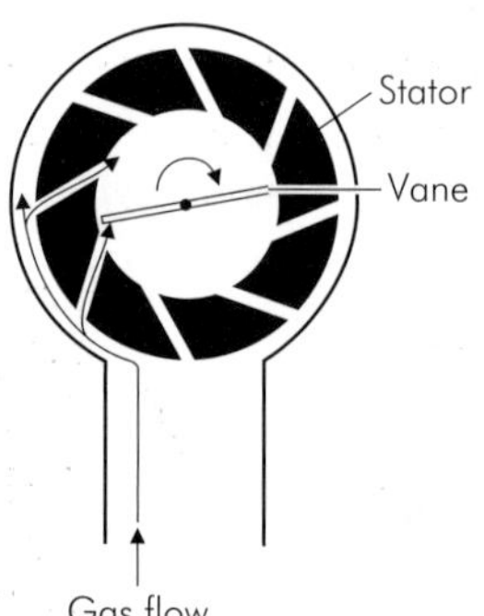

Figure 8.7 *Cross-section of a Wright respirometer*

What are the advantages and disadvantages of Wright's respirometer?
The advantage is that it is small and portable and requires no power supply.

It only measures the flow in one direction. Its accuracy varies with the flow. It over-reads at high flow rate and under reads at low flow rate. Water condensation from the expired gases can cause the pointer to stick and adds inertia.

What is the principle of the pneumotachograph?
It is a 'constant resistance, variable pressure' type of flowmeter. $Q = P/R$. As the resistance is constant any change in pressure is directly proportional to the flow.

It consists of a tube with a fixed resistance. As the gas flows through the fixed resistance there will be a pressure drop. A differential pressure transducer senses the pressure gradient across the resistance. The pressure change is proportional to the flow.

What factors can affect the pressure gradient?

The pressure gradient is dependent on the flow rate, density and viscosity and temperature of the gas mixture. Condensation of moisture increases the screen resistance and may cause turbulence. In modern pneumotachographs there is a heater incorporated to avoid water condensation.

Do you know the various types of pneumotachographs and how do they work?

- Screen pneumotachograph.
- Fleisch pneumotachograph.
- Hot-wire pneumotachograph.
- Pitot tube.

A screen pneumotachograph consists of a short connector with a gauze screen mounted across the middle, through which the gas flows. The measuring head has a sufficiently large diameter to ensure laminar flow. The screen acts as a flow resistance and produces a small pressure drop across it. There are two pressure-sampling ports on either side of the screen which feed differential pressure to a differential pressure transducer (Figure 8.8a).

The Fleisch pneumotachograph head consists of a bundle of fine bore parallel tubes which provides a linear flow resistance. It is larger and bulkier than the screen

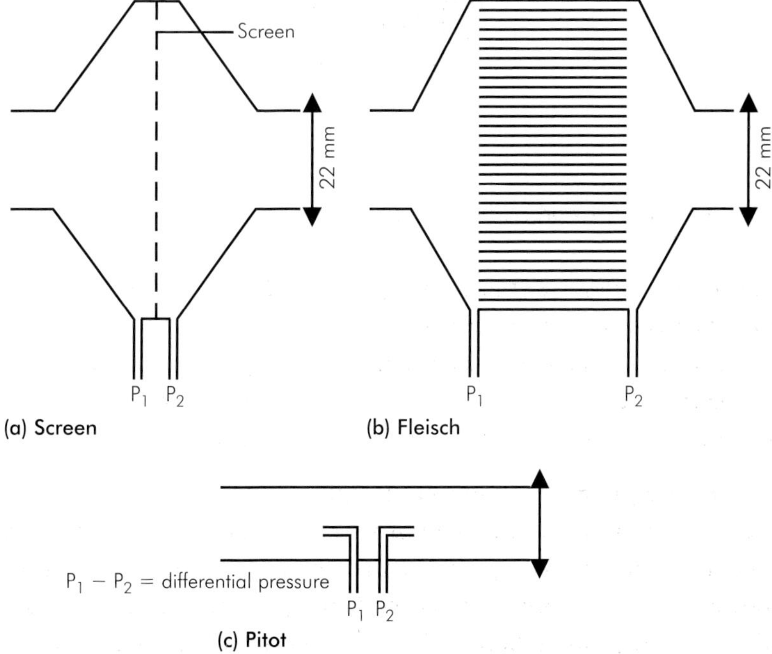

Figure 8.8 *Pneumotachograph heads*

head. Water vapour condensation can be avoided by heating the parallel tubes (Figure 8.8b).

A hot wire pneumotachograph has two hot wires mounted at right angles to each other across the lumen of the pneumotachograph head. The gas flow produces cooling of the wires which is dependent on the flow rate.

A pitot tube flow meter consists of a connector with two small diameter sampling tube mounted axially in the centre of a gas flow path. The open ends of these tubes act as pressure sampling ports. One sampling port faces upstream and other faces downstream. The upstream port measures a higher pressure due to the impact of gas and other port measures a static pressure. The difference between these two pressure ports is measured by differential pressure transducer. Advantages of the pitot tube are, it is simple, small in size and less dead space (Figure 8.8c).

Do the pneumotachographs measure the tidal volume directly?

No, they measure the flow. Tidal volume is calculated by integrating flow over inspiratory or expiratory time.

SOE 9

Physiology 9

Key topics: protein metabolism, adrenal hormones, respiratory system compliance

Q1 Protein metabolism

What is the structure of a protein?

Amino acids form the basic units of proteins. Each amino acid has a carboxyl group (COOH) and amine group (NH_2) attached to a carbon atom. Chains of amino acids are called peptides or polypeptides. These chains increase in size to form proteins.

What are glycoproteins and lipoproteins?

These are proteins containing carbohydrates and lipids respectively.

What you mean by essential amino acids? Can you name some essential aminoacids?

Those amino acids that are not synthesised endogenously and are dependent on dietary source alone are called essential amino acids:

- Methionine, arginine, threonine, tryptophan.
- Valine, isoleucine, leucine.
- Phenylalanine, lysine.

What are the metabolic functions of amino acids?

- Protein synthesis.
- Several hormones, catecholamines and neurotransmitters are formed from specific amino acids. Methionine, for example, is converted to S-adenosyl methionine, which is an active methylating agent in the synthesis of epinephrine.

- Fatty acid synthesis.
- Gluconeogenesis.
- Citric acid cycle.
- Transamination.
- Precursors for purines and pyrimidines.

What is the function of purines and pyrimidines?

These ring based structures are ubiquitous in the body and are the base components in the ribonucleotides and deoxyribonucleotides that code RNA and DNA respectively.

Purines and pyrimidines contain high-energy phosphoryl bonds which are involved in several phosphate transfer reactions of ATP and other nucleoside triphosphates (GTP, UTP).

They also form coenzymes such as coenzyme A, $NADP^+$ and NAD^+.

Can you name some ketogenic aminoacids? Why are they so called?

Leucine, isoleucine and tyrosine are ketogenic aminoacids as they can be converted to the ketone body, acetoacetate.

How is urea formed? Tell me about urea cycle.

Ammonia is the end product of amino acid metabolism. The amino acids are deaminated to release NH_4^+. Two organs play important role in handling ammonia, the kidneys and the liver. In the kidneys, NH_4^+ dissociates into NH_3 and H^+ and is excreted in urine. In the liver, ammonia is converted to and eliminated as urea.

In the urea cycle, ammonia combines with carbon dioxide to form carbamyl phosphate. Inside the mitochondria it is transformed into ornithine, then to citrulline.

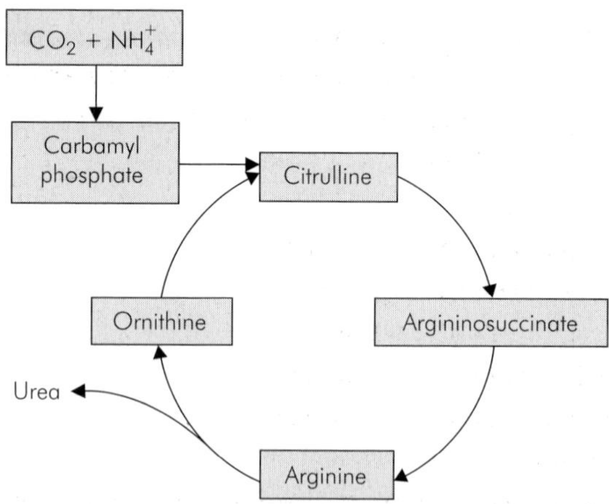

Figure 9.1 *Urea cycle*

Citrulline is converted to arginine which splits into urea and ornithine. Ornithine re-enters the cycle.

Can you tell me about the synthesis of creatine and creatinine? Why are they important?

Creatine is synthesised in the liver from methionine, glycine and arginine. It is present in muscle, brain and blood. Creatine has high-energy phosphoryl bonds. This is important in generating the ATP necessary to provide energy for initial phase of muscle contraction. The phosphorylation of creatine is facilitated by the enzyme creatine kinase. This enzyme is used as a marker of degree of skeletal muscle damage following trauma or cardiac muscle damage following myocardial infarction.

Creatinine is formed in muscle. It is the anhydride form of creatine and is a metabolite which is excreted in the urine. Creatinine excretion in the urine is proportional to total muscle mass.

Q2 Adrenal gland

What are the hormones produced by the adrenal cortex?

The three main types of steroid hormones released from the adrenal cortex include mineralocorticoids, glucocorticoids and androgens.

The adrenal cortex has three zones (*GFR as a mnemonic*):

- Zona **G**lomerulosa secretes aldosterone, the mineralocorticoid.
- Zona **F**asciculata secretes cortisol, the glucocorticoid.
- Zona **R**eticulosa secretes androgens.

What are the effects of glucocorticoids?

- *Metabolic effects*:
  - Protein and carbohydrate metabolism.
  - Increase in hepatic gluconeogenesis and glycogen deposition.
  - Inhibition of glucose uptake in muscle and adipose tissue.
  - Lypolysis in adipose tissue.
  - Protein catabolism.
- *Effect on immune and inflammatory response*:
  - Inhibition of prostaglandin synthesis.
  - Suppression of lymphokine release.
  - Decrease in the synthesis of IgG and IgE.
  - Modulation and function of leucocytes.
- *Mineralocorticoid effects*:
  - Promotes retention of sodium, chloride and water in exchange for potassium and hydrogen ion elimination.

- *Permissive effects*:
  - Insulin and catecholamines require the presence of glucocorticoids to exert their effect. In particular, during stress, the cardiovascular effects of catecholamines are blunted in the absence of glucocorticoids.

Can you explain the feedback control of glucocorticoid secretion?

Adrenocorticotrophic hormone (ACTH) from the anterior pituitary is the most important stimulus for the secretion of cortisol. This ACTH is in turn controlled by corticotrophin releasing hormone (CRH) from the hypothalamus. Cortisol inhibits both ACTH and CRH thereby providing a negative feedback control.

There is a normal circadian pattern whereby 75% of the daily production of ACTH occurs between 4 a.m. and 10 a.m. Cortisol level peaks in the mornings.

Trauma, emotion and stress stimulate CRH release.

What is the basic structure of adrenocortical harmones?

The basic structure is a steroid nucleus. The precursor of all corticosteroids is cholesterol.

Can you draw the structure of a steroid nucleus?

Cyclo-pentano-perhydro-phenanthrene nucleus.

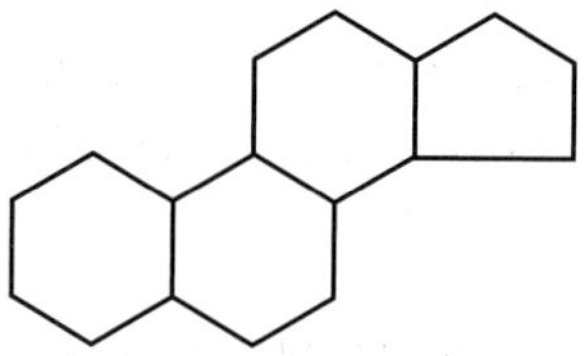

Figure 9.2 *Steroid nucleus*

Can you take me through the pathway involved in the synthesis of the adrenocortical hormones?

As in Diagram (Figure 9.3).

What is the mechanism of action of ACTH?

ACTH binds to the receptors on the membrane of adrenocortical cells. This activates adenyl cyclase which causes an increase in cyclic AMP. As a result there is activation of protein kinase A, which phosphorylates cholesterol ester hydrolase. Cholesterol esters are converted to free cholesterol. Cholesterol is the precursor for the steroid hormones.

What are the effects of aldosterone?

The important actions of aldosterone concern sodium and potassium balance. In the distal renal tubules aldosterone causes active reabsorption of sodium by increasing

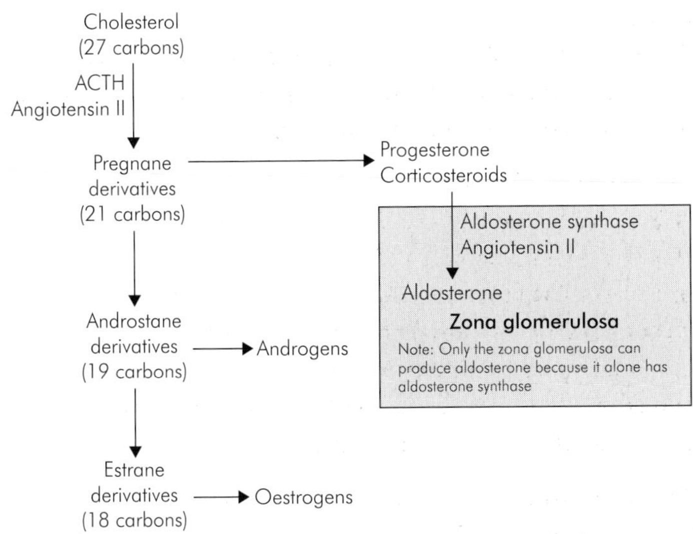

Figure 9.3 *Synthesis of cortical hormones*

the activity of NA^+K^+ ATPase pump. There is a passive reabsorption of water along with sodium thereby increasing the extracellular fluid volume.

Aldosterone stimulates active excretion of potassium from the distal tubular cells. Aldosterone also has action on other organs in the body involving sodium transport, as in the gastrointestinal tract.

Can you explain the feedback control of aldosterone secretion?

Decrease in extracellular fluid (ECF) volume, decrease in renal perfusion pressure, or a fall in serum sodium concentration cause activation of the renin–angiotensin system. This results in an increase in angiotensin II that acts on the zona glomerulosa to cause increased synthesis and release of aldosterone.

An increase in plasma potassium concentration is also an important stimulus of aldosterone secretion. ACTH does not play an important role in controlling aldosterone secretion.

Q3 Respiratory system compliance

Define compliance.

Compliance is a change in volume for a given unit change in pressure. In respiratory system this describes the 'ease with which the lungs can expand'.

What are the two major components influencing total respiratory compliance?

They are the lung compliance and the chest wall compliance.

Can you draw a graph demonstrating the compliance of the respiratory system?

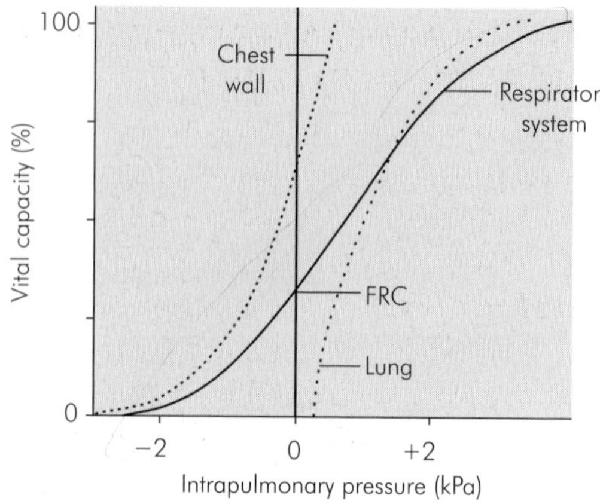

Figure 9.4 *Lung and chest wall compliance*

The x-axis relates to the pressure change (intrapulmonary pressure) and the y-axis the volume change (vital capacity). The curve is almost linear in the working range around functional residual capacity (FRC). At higher volumes the muscle fibres are already fully stretched and hence the compliance reduces. At lower volumes the airway and alveolar collapse occurs. Therefore more pressure is required to open them, a lower compliance.

What is the normal intrapleural pressure?

At FRC, when the lungs and the chest wall are in relative resting stage, the intrapleural pressure is about −0.3 kPa. During quiet inspiration this reduces further to −1.0 kPa. With forced inspiration it can go as negative as −4.0 kPa.

What is the difference between static and dynamic compliance?

Essentially they represent different measurement techniques. When measuring static compliance, after applying a known distending pressure, adequate time is allowed for the gas to equilibrate in the lung and then the change in the volume is measured.

On the other hand, when measuring dynamic compliance, the changes in volume and pressure are recorded continuously during spontaneous breathing or mechanical ventilation without giving any time pause for the equilibration.

For a given lung volume, the airway pressure will always be higher in a dynamic environment than those in the static case. Compliance is change in volume/change in pressure and therefore because of higher pressures dynamic compliance will always be less than the static compliance.

What is hysteresis?

When the pressure–volume curve is plotted both during inspiration and expiration the curve does not follow the same tracing but rather forms a loop where the return path differs from the first. This is known as 'hysteresis'.

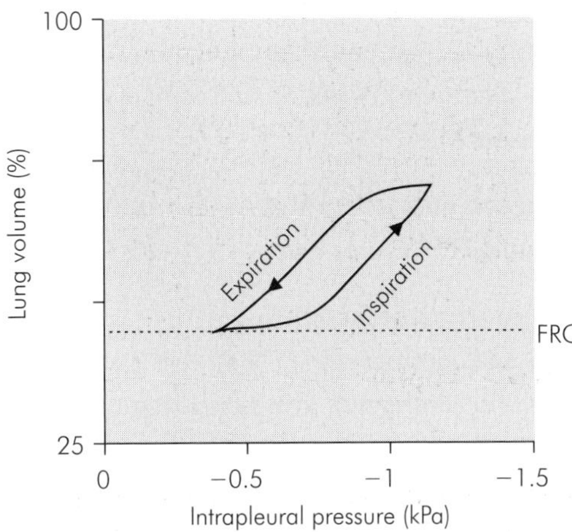

Figure 9.5 *Inspiration–expiration loop showing hysteresis*

The area within the loop represents the energy expended during the work of breathing. This wasted energy is spent on stretching and recoil of tissues (viscous losses) and to overcome airway resistance (frictional losses).

Pharmacology 9

Key topics: MAC, xenon, drug interaction, antibiotics

Q1 Minimum alveolar concentration

Can you define MAC?

MAC is defined as minimum alveolar concentration of an agent in oxygen at a steady state that prevents movement in response to a standard surgical stimulation (surgical incision) in 50% of subjects at atmospheric pressure.

What is the clinical use of MAC?

MAC of an agent is used to compare the potency of volatile anaesthetic agents.

What factors can affect MAC?

- *Physiological factors*: At infancy and childhood MAC is high, with increasing age MAC value decreases. Pregnancy reduces the MAC.
- *Metabolic factors*: Hypothermia and hypothyroidism will reduce the MAC whereas hyperthermia and hyperthyroidism will increase the MAC.
- *Pharmacological factors*: Premedication with benzodiazepines will reduce the MAC. Clonidine, lithium, α adrenoreceptor agonists and opioid analgesics will reduce MAC. Acute alcohol intoxication will reduce the MAC whereas chronic alcohol intake increases MAC.

Can you name some agents with a very high MAC value?

Nitrous oxide-105, Xenon-71.

What are the physical properties of xenon?

It is an inert, colourless and odourless gas. It has a very low blood/gas solubility (0.14) giving rapid induction and elimination. It is non-irritant to the respiratory tract. Its molecular weight is 131.2 Da and it has a boiling point of 108°C. It is compatible with soda lime. It is non-flammable and does not support combustion.

Tell me about the pharmacodynamic properties of xenon?

The central nervous system effects are readily reversible and there is no stimulant activity. It produces unconsciousness with analgesia and a degree of muscle relaxation at concentrations above 60%. Cerebral blood flow is increased. It is very cardiostable and does not sensitise myocardium to catecholamines. It has no long-term adverse effects with chronic exposure at low dose.

Q2 Drug interactions

What do you understand by drug interaction?

Drug interaction is the modification of the effects of one drug by another. This interaction may increase or decrease the action of the second drug. Some interactions are beneficial and can be used in clinical practice where as some interactions may result in unwanted effects.

How do you classify drug interactions? Can you give me some examples?

- *Physicochemical.*
- *Pharmacodynamic*: Receptor based or enzyme based.
- *Pharmacokinetic*: Absorption, metabolism, excretion and protein binding.

What do you mean by physiochemical interactions?

Physicochemical interactions are caused by chemical or physical incompatibility between the preparations used. This may result in loss of activity of the drug or precipitation of the drugs. For example, thiopental and suxamethonium precipitate when mixed in the same syringe.

What is the cause of physical incompatibility?

A change in pH of a solution caused by mixing can result in drug precipitation. Midazolam hydrochloride is a salt of a weak base and a strong acid. As the pH of the solution increases its solubility decreases.

What are pharmacodynamic interactions?

These interactions occur as a result of competition for the binding site of an enzyme or receptor. These interactions can be direct when the drugs act on the same receptor system or indirect when two drugs produce the same effect by different mechanisms.

For example, flumazenil is a competitive antagonist to midazolam and reverses the clinical effects of midazolam (direct interaction). Neostigmine inhibits acetyl cholinesterase and increases the concentration of acetylcholine and displaces atracurium from the nicotinic receptors (indirect interaction). Pharmacodynamic interactions can produce additive, synergistic or antagonistic effects depending on the affinity and efficacy of the agent involved.

Can you give some examples of pharmacokinetic interactions?

These interactions occur due to the effects of co-administered drugs on absorption, distribution, metabolism and elimination.

- *Absorption*: The combination of iron and tetracycline in the stomach significantly impair the absorption of both drugs. Addition of epinephrine to local anaesthetic solution reduces the systemic absorption and prolongs the duration of the local anaesthetic. Metoclopramide decreases gastric emptying time and promotes absorption of other co-administered drugs.
- *Protein binding*: Competition for protein binding sites on plasma proteins may result in displacement of initial drug by the newer drug. Sulphonamides displace warfarin from their binding sites and increase the free warfarin level.
- *Drug distribution*: Beta blockers reduce the cardiac output and may reduce the distribution of other drugs to their site of action.
- *Metabolism*: Drugs can interfere with a single common metabolic pathway or interfere with enzymatic processes. Drugs such as phenytoin, rifampicin, ethanol and barbiturates induce higher levels of hepatic microsomal enzyme activity which accelerate their metabolism.

  In contrast cimetidine reversibly binds to cytochrome P_{450} enzyme and inhibits drug metabolism.
- *Excretion*: Renal excretion may be affected by mechanical means by increasing or decreasing urine output. Sodium bicarbonate will make the urine more

alkaline and enhance the excretion of weak acids such as barbiturates or aspirin.

Can you explain the interaction between opioids and monoamino oxidase inhibitors?
There are two types of interactions that can occur particularly with pethidine.

- *Excitatory form*: This is characterised by agitation, delirium, headache, hypertension, rigidity, hyperpyrexia and coma. This type of interaction is only seen in patients receiving pethidine or dextramorphan. This is probably due to increased concentrations of 5 hydroxy tryptamine (serotonin) in the central nervous system. Mono-amino oxidase inhibitor (MAOI) prevents the break down of 5-HT. Pethidine blocks the uptake of 5-HT. Hence the concentration of 5-HT will be substantially increased.
- *Depressive form*: This is characterised by severe cardiovascular and respiratory depression and coma. This situation is probably due to inhibition of hepatic microsomal enzymes by MAOIs resulting in an accumulation of pethidine.

Q3 Antibiotics

What do you understand by the term antibiotic?
An antibiotic is a chemical substance that is produced by microorganisms and has the capacity to kill or inhibit the growth of another microorganism.

What you mean by bacteriostatic and bactericidal?
Bacteriostatic antibiotics prevent the growth of bacteria and bactericidal ones kill the bacteria.

Can you name some beta-lactam antibiotics?
Penicillins (benzyl penicillin, amoxycillin, flucloxacillin), cephalosporins, monobactams and carbapenems.

Why are they called β-lactams?
Their structure contains β-lactam ring and hence they are called β-lactams.

What is their mechanism of action?
They inhibit the cell wall synthesis by binding to various proteins on the bacterial cell wall. The bacterial cell wall is weakened and lysis occurs.

How does resistance develop? What is the mechanism?
Bacteria exhibit resistance to β-lactam antibiotics by following mechanisms.

- Bacteria produce a β-lactamase enzyme that hydrolysis the β-lactam ring.
- Bacteria modify their cell wall proteins so that antibiotic cannot bind to the specific protein.
- The cell wall can become impermeable to antibiotics.

Do you know a β-lactamase inhibitor that is used together with an antibiotic?
Clavulanic acid is used in combination with amoxycillin to improve the antibacterial activity.

Please name some cephalosporins.

- *First-generation cephalosporins*: cephazolin and cepharadine. These are active against β-lactamase producing staphylococci.
- *Second-generation cephalosporins*: cephalexin, cefaclor and cefuroxime. These are more resistant to β-lactamase.
- *Third-generation cephalosporins* these have improved Gram-negative activity – cefotaxime, ceftriaxone, ceftazidime.
- *Fourth-generation cephalosporins*: cefpirome.

Do you know any other mechanisms by which antibiotics act?
Some antibiotics can inhibit bacterial protein synthesis and some can inhibit the synthesis of nucleic acid.

- *Inhibition of protein synthesis*:
  - Aminoglycosides bind to the bacterial ribosomal RNA subunit and block the protein synthesis (e.g. gentamicin, netilmicin and tobramycin).
  - Macrolides (erythromycin and azithromycin) also block the protein synthesis by binding to the ribosomal subunit of RNA.
- *Inhibition of nucleic acid synthesis*:
  - Quinolones (nalidixic acid, ciprofloxacin, norfloxacin and oflaxacin) inhibit the alpha-subunit of the DNA-gyrase enzyme.
  - Rifampicin binds to the DNA-dependent RNA polymerase and prevents the transcription of DNA into RNA.

Where do we use vancomycin?
Often in intensive care. Vancomycin is commonly used to treat methicillin-resistant *Staphylococcus aureus* (MRSA). It is a glycopeptide active against most Gram-positive bacteria, coagulase-negative staphylococci and Gram-positive anaerobes such as clostridia.

What is the mechanism of action?
It is a bactericidal antimicrobial that inhibits the glycopeptide synthetase and prevents formation of peptidoglycan in the bacterial cell wall.

What are the side effects of vancomycin?
Nephrotoxicity is rare, usually seen when administered with other antibiotics causing nephrotoxicity or in the presence of pre-existing renal impairment.

Ototoxicity can also occur in the presence of another ototoxic drug and or with pre-existing renal impairment.

Rapid intravenous administration can cause histamine release resulting in hypotension, tachycardia and rashes.

Phlebitis can occur if administered undiluted.

Clinical 9

Key topics: squint, paediatric anaesthesia, bradycardia, suxamethonium apnoea

Q1 A 3-year-old child is scheduled for correction of a squint in the left eye as a day case procedure

Describe the preoperative assessment of this child?

Take a detailed history from the parents about the child's general health, any previous anaesthetics, current medications and allergies and family history of any anaesthetic problems. Ask about normal milestones and development. Immunisation history may be helpful.

What family history are you particularly concerned about?

Squint can be a part of generalised muscle disorder. Patients with these muscle disorders can have a predisposition to malignant hyperthermia. When assessing patients with a squint it is important to elicit any family history suggestive of malignant hyperthermia in any of the family members.

What muscle disorders have an association with malignant hyperthermia?

A muscle disorder with a strong association with malignant hyperthermia is central core disease, an inherited disorder characterised by peripheral muscle weakness. Other possible conditions include myotonia congenita and the Duchenne type of muscular dystrophy.

How long do you want this child to be starved before the operation?

2 h for clear liquids, 4 h for milk, 6 h for solids.

Will you administer any premedication?

Topical local anaesthetic such as eutectic mixture of local anaesthetics (EMLA) or amethocaine is useful for painless intravenous cannulation. In an uncooperative child sedation may be given. Oral midazolam 0.4–0.5 mg/kg about 15 min before the operation can be used. Oral atropine 20 μg/kg is sometimes used for its vagolytic effect and reduction of secretions. Preoperative analgesia can be provided with soluble paracetamol 20 mg/kg orally.

What are the basic differences between a child and adult?

Children are different from adults physically, physiologically and psychologically.

- *Airway and Breathing*: Children are obligatory nose breathers, hence maintaining patency of the nasal air passages is important. Infants have a large head, large tongue, short neck and a small mouth. The epiglottis is floppy and U shaped. The larynx is positioned higher than adult (at the level of C4 in a child, C5 in an adult). The narrowest part of the airway is at the level of cricoid in children whereas in adults it is at the level of vocal cords. The trachea is short and this predisposes endobronchial intubation. Infants have a limited ability to increase tidal volume because of a horizontal rib cage. In adults the bucket handle effect of the rib cage allows a significant increase in the anteroposterior diameter. Children have a more compliant chest wall and relatively low functional residual capacity. Basal oxygen consumption is 2–3 times higher in children.
- *Circulation*: Children have a limited ability to increase stroke volume because of stiffer ventricles. The cardiac output is therefore mainly dependent on heart rate (HR). Their parasympathetic nervous system is well developed and hence often the first manifestation of several physiological insults can be bradycardia rather than tachycardia.
- *Renal*: Renal blood flow and glomerular filtration rate is low in first 2 years of life. Both fluid overload and dehydration are poorly tolerated in young children.
- *Temperature control*: Children have large surface area:weight ratio. The shivering mechanism is poorly developed.

What are the specific problems in anaesthetising a 3-year-old child?

- *Preoperative*: Children may be emotionally upset because of the hospital environment and may not be co-operative with clinical examination.
- *Induction*: Children may be uncooperative during induction and pre-oxygenation is usually not possible. Intravenous access can be difficult and this dictates gas induction. Due to lack of preoxygenation, reduced functional residual capacity (FRC) and high metabolic rate they can rapidly desaturate.

Laryngoscopy and tracheal intubation can be difficult in small children.

- *Anaesthetic equipment*: Breathing systems and airway devices are specific. Drug dosages should be pre-calculated.
- *Monitoring*: Children may not be co-operative for attaching the monitoring devices like electrocardiogram (ECG), non-invasive blood pressure (NIBP) and pulse oximeter before induction. Failure to choose the appropriate size cuffs can lead to erroneous blood pressure (BP) reading. In addition, they require special paediatric pulse oximeter probes.

- *Recovery and extubation*: As for induction, appropriate monitoring and oxygen administration is difficult. Children are more likely to suffer airway complications such as laryngeal oedema and laryngospasm.

What are the basic requirements of a breathing system for paediatric use?

- Low dead space.
- Low resistance.
- Lightweight.
- Reliable for providing adequate oxygenation and elimination of carbon dioxide.

What is the estimated weight of this 3-year-old child?

A suitable formula is: (age + 4) × 2 = 14 kg.

What is the normal HR and BP at this age?

HR = 90–110/min, BP = 90–100 mmHg systolic (80 + age × 2); 50–60 mmHg diastolic.

How will you anaesthetise this child?

Preoperative visit and explanation to the parents. Consent for suppository analgesia.

Induction may be inhalational or intravenous. Monitoring to minimum standards, Glycopyrrolate 10 μg/kg at induction. Laryngeal mask airway (LMA) or endotracheal tube (ETT).

Avoid suxamethonium as it can cause tonic contraction of extra-ocular muscles, which can last upto 20 min, making the surgery difficult.

General anaesthesia with spontaneous or controlled ventilation. For analgesia, intravenous fentanyl, paracetamol or diclofenac suppository. Maintenance with oxygen + air/N_2O + volatile or propofol infusion.

What size ETT will you use for this child?

A suitable formula is: 4 + age/4 = mm of ID = 5 mm ETT and 12 + Age/2 = 13.5 cm length at lip.

Do you use a cuffed tube? Why not?

A plain ETT should be used in children less than 10-years old. For a given size a cuffed tube will have a larger outer circumference at the level of cuff. Halving the diameter will increase the resistance by 16 times. As cricoid is the narrowest part, an inflated cuff can cause mucosal damage at this level. This can cause laryngeal oedema.

Can you use an LMA?

Yes. Access to the airway is limited during intraoperative period. The anaesthetic machine is away from the airway. While using the microscope surgeon requires an immobile surgical field. None of these preclude LMA use.

What size LMA will you choose for this child?

A size 2 is suitable.

How will you decide the appropriate size of LMA and how much air do you need to inflate for an adequate seal?

Table 9.1 *LMA sizes*

Patient weight (kg)	<5	5–10	10–20	20–30	30–50	50–70	70–100
LMA size	1	1½	2	2½	3	4	5
Maximum inflation volume	4 ml	7 ml	10 ml	14 ml	20 ml	30 ml	40 ml

What are the benefits of using an LMA?

- Muscle relaxants can be avoided.
- The problems associated with laryngoscopy and intubation can be minimised.
- Sympatho-adrenal response is less.
- Recovery phase is smooth with fewer incidences of airway problems in recovery.

How do you calculate the maintenance fluid requirement in children?

Maintenance fluid in paediatric practice is calculated with the rule of 4:2:1. For the first 10 kg–4 ml/kg/hour; the second 10 kg–2 ml/kg/hour and every subsequent kg–1 ml/kg/hour. For example, this child weighs about 14 kg. So the maintenance fluid will be

$(10 \times 4\,\text{ml}) = 40\,\text{ml} + (4 \times 2\,\text{ml}) = 8\,\text{ml}.$

This makes 48 ml/hour.

What will be the blood volume in a 3-year-old child?

$80\,\text{ml/kg} = 80 \times 14 = 1120\,\text{ml}.$

Q2 Critical incident: bradycardia

Let us return to the squint operation. While half way through the operation, you notice that the ECG rate is 50 per minute. How will you proceed?

Quickly confirm the rate, check pulse oximeter trace.

Check the airway, administer 100% oxygen. Inform the surgeon, stop the procedure. In the mean time if these measures fail to restore the normal HR, call for senior help.

Atropine 20 μg/kg or glycopyrrolate 10 μg/kg intravenous should be given. Cardiopulmonary resuscitation (CPR) must be considered if cardiac output is lost.

What may have caused this event?

Intraoperative bradycardia can be due to anaesthetic factors, surgical factors or patient factors.

- *Anaesthetic factors*: Hypoxia, drugs such as halothane, opioids and propofol.
- *Surgical factors*: Stimulating structures with parasympathetic innervation, traction on the extra-ocular muscles for example.
- *Patient factors*: Hypothermia, cardiac conduction defects, endocrine abnormalities. In this case the most likely cause is due to the stretch of extra-ocular muscles, in particular the medial rectus resulting in the oculo-cardiac reflex.

What is the mechanism for the oculo-cardiac reflex?

Following stretch of extra-ocular muscles afferent impulses travel via the ciliary ganglion through the ophthalmic division of the trigeminal nerve. They are thence transmitted to the Gasserian ganglion and finally reach the sensory nucleus of trigeminal nerve.

Efferent impulses pass through the vagus nerve.

What other arrhythmias may be seen during squint surgery?

The other arrhythmias can be junctional rhythm, atrial ectopics, bigeminy and ventricular tachycardia.

How can these be prevented?

Gentle traction during surgery. Prophylactic use of vagolytics (glycopyrrolate or atropine) has been shown to reduce the incidence of oculocardiac reflex.

How will you manage intraoperative and postoperative analgesia?

Fentanyl 1–2 μg/kg intravenously should be adequate for intraoperative analgesia.

Paracetamol in an initial dose of 20–40 mg/kg; diclofenac: 1–1.5 mg/kg in the form of suppositories are effective way to keep the child comfortable in the immediate postoperative period. Topical local anaesthesia with amethocaine helps in supplementing analgesia.

What is the incidence of postoperative nausea and vomiting (PONV) in squint surgery?

It is very high and can exceed 50%.

How do you prevent it?

- Careful and gentle mask ventilation during induction to avoid gastric insufflation.
- Prophylaxis with ondansetron 0.1 mg/kg; dexamethasone 0.1 mg/kg.
- Adequate hydration.
- Avoiding long acting opioids.

Q3 Suxamethonium apnoea

You have anaesthetised a 20-year-old male patient for appendicectomy. At the end of operation after reversal of neuromuscular block, he fails to breath. How do you manage this patient?

Use an Airway Breathing and Circulation (ABC) approach.

Continue ventilation and monitoring. Check the anaesthetic chart for timing of opioid and muscle relaxants administration, meanwhile assess and investigate for possible causes.

What are the possible causes?

- Drugs. Muscle relaxants – inadequate reversal of neuromuscular block, suxamethonium apnoea. Relative or absolute overdose of opioids and benzodiazepines.
- Hypothermia.
- Electrolyte imbalance – hypokalaemia, hypermagnesaemia.
- Hyperglycaemia, hypoglycaemia, hypothyroidism.
- Cerebrovascular accident or neuromuscular disorders brought to light by an abnormal response to anaesthesia.

How can you diagnose suxamethonium apnoea?

Suspect it on clinical grounds where suxamethonium has been administered and other possible causes have been excluded. Neuromuscular monitoring with train of four may reveal reduction in height of all four twitches, no fade with tetanic stimulation and no post-tetanic facilitation.

How do you manage suxamethonium apnoea?

Continue sedation and support ventilation until the neuromuscular block wears off.

What tests do you need to do to confirm suxamethonium apnoea? When will you do?

Take a blood sample from the patient and request dibucaine number and serum cholinesterase level. Wait at least 3 days after exposure to suxamethonium before testing.

Wait at least 8 weeks after homologous blood transfusion before testing.

What does the dibucaine number tell you?

The dibucaine number is the percentage inhibition of plasma cholinesterase by the amide local anaesthetic, dibucaine. Normal value is 75–85%. A number less than 20 indicates homozygous variant of abnormal cholinesterase.

What is the normal level of plasma cholinesterase?

It is 1000–3500 units/l.

Physics, clinical measurement and safety 9

Key topics: oxygen measurement, heat loss, electrocardiogram

Q1 Oxygen measurement

How can you measure F_IO_2 in a gas mixture?

The concentration of oxygen in a gas mixture can be measured using following methods:

- Galvanic fuel cell.
- Clark polarographic electrode.
- Paramagnetic analyser.
- Mass spectrometer.

What is the principle of the fuel cell?

It consists of a gold or silver cathode, lead anode and potassium bicarbonate buffer solution. At the anode hydroxyl ions from potassium hydroxide solution combine with lead to produce electrons. Oxygen molecules diffuse through the membrane and combine with the electrons and water at the cathode to give hydroxyl ions. This process generates a current which is proportional to the partial pressure of oxygen. If more oxygen is available more electrons will be taken up by the cathode. A fuel cell

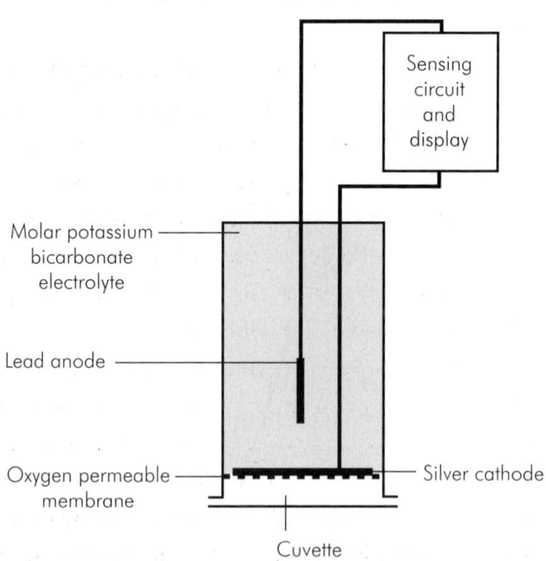

Figure 9.6 *Galvanic fuel cell*

produces a voltage and hence acts as a battery. Like any other batteries it has a shelf life which depends on the duration of exposure to oxygen. The reaction is:

$$Pb + 2OH^- \rightarrow PbO + 2H_2O + 2e^-$$
$$O_2 + e^- + 2H_2O \rightarrow 4OH^-$$

A fuel cell is compact and does not require power supply. It is not affected by nitrous oxide.

What are the disadvantages of a fuel cell?
It has a relatively slow response time of around 20 s. It cannot measure breath-to-breath changes. Life span is limited to 6–12 months.

How do you calibrate a fuel cell?
It is calibrated for 21% exposing it to room air and then to 100% oxygen.

What is the principle employed in a paramagnetic oxygen analyser?
Oxygen contains two unpaired electrons in the outermost orbit and hence it is attracted towards a magnetic field. Substances attracted by the magnetic field are known as paramagnetic and the substances repelled by the magnetic field are known as diamagnetic. Nitrogen and most gases used in anaesthesia are weakly diamagnetic and are repelled from a magnetic field.

Do you know any different types of paramagnetic analyser?
How do they work?
The Pauling paramagnetic analyser is an older simple version. Various modifications have been made to the basic design to compensate for external vibration, excessive gas-flow rate and pressurisation of the cell. These are null-deflection type paramagnetic analyser and pulsed-field paramagnetic analyser.

The Pauling type of paramagnetic analyser consists of two glass spheres filled with nitrogen. These are connected in a dumbell arrangement and placed in a non-uniform magnetic field in gas tight chamber by suspending on a filament. There is a mirror which is attached to the dumbell.

The gas sample containing oxygen is delivered to the chamber. The paramagnetic effect of oxygen displaces the glass spheres and the dumbell rotates until the force of this displacement is balanced by the tension of the filament. As the dumbell rotates the mirror also rotates. A light beam is passed to the mirror and the reflected beam is detected by a photocell detector which measures the degree of rotation. The degree of rotation is proportional to the concentration of oxygen in the chamber.

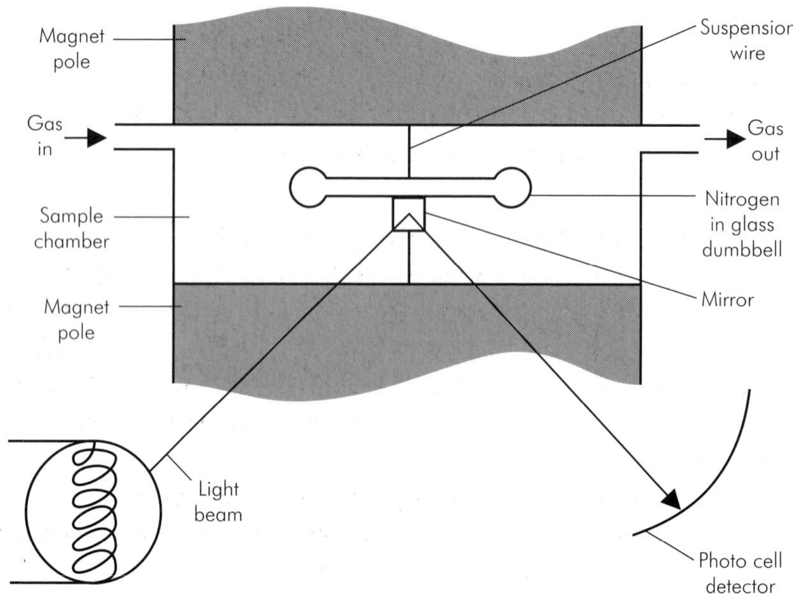

Figure 9.7 *Pauling type of paramagnetic analyser*

In the null deflection type paramagnetic analyser, reflected light is detected by the photo-detector cells. Output from these cells is used to generate current flow. This current flows around the dumbell and is used to produce an opposing magnetic field that maintains the dumbell in a neutral position. The current required to keep the dumbell in a neutral position is a measure of oxygen concentration. This system is more accurate than the Pauling paramagnetic analyser.

In a pulsed-field para-magnetic analyser reference (room air) and sample gas are delivered as separate streams to a magnetic field. These two streams are separated by a pressure sensitive transducer. A magnet is rapidly switched on and off creating a pulsed magnetic field. When the magnet is switched on the stream containing more oxygen is attracted to the magnetic field and this produces a pressure difference across the transducer. The pressure difference across the transducer is proportional to the O_2 partial pressure difference between the sample and reference gases.

The newer versions of paramagnetic analysers are very accurate and highly sensitive. They have a rapid response time allowing breath-to-breath oxygen analysis. Hence both the inspired and expired oxygen concentrations can be measured. Water vapour can affect the performance, hence the sample gases are dried by passing through silica gel before entering the analysis cell.

Q2 Heat loss

What happens to body temperature under general anaesthesia?
Under general anaesthesia and in the operating theatre due to various mechanisms, heat loss is increased and body temperature is reduced.

What mechanisms contribute to reduced body temperature?
General anaesthesia depresses the thermoregulatory centre and many anaesthetic agents have an effect on the vasomotor centre reducing the vasomotor tone. There is peripheral vasodilatation which increases the heat loss. Other factors related to surgery and anaesthesia such as exposure of body cavity, irrigation of cold fluids, operating room temperature and infusion of cold fluids will also contribute to hypothermia.

The principle routes of heat loss during anaesthesia and surgery are:

- *Conduction*: Heat loss is due to direct contact with another object which is at lower temperature such as the operating table.
- *Radiation*: Heat loss by infrared radiation from the exposed portions of the body to the neighbouring objects which are not in direct contact. This may account for about 40% of total heat loss.
- *Convection*: The air layer adjacent to the surface of body is warmed as it expands and thus becomes less dense and rises. This produces a convection current which carries heat away from the subject. These currents will be further increased by the added effect of laminar flow in the operating theatre.
- *Evaporation*: Evaporation of sweat from the skin or body fluids from mucosal or tissue surfaces results in heat loss due to the latent heat of evaporation.
- *Respiration*: This accounts for about 10% of heat loss. Inspiration of dry gases increases the heat loss from respiration.

(Mnemonic – **R**oyal **C**ollege **E**xam **R**oom, **R**adiation: 40%; **C**onvection: 30%; **E**vaporation: 20%; **R**espiration: 10%).

What measures can be used to prevent hypothermia?

- Heat loss by radiation can be reduced by increasing the room temperature and covering exposed surfaces with warm blankets.
- Heat loss by respiration can be minimised humidifying the inspired gases. Intravenous fluids should be warmed during infusion.
- Warm fluids should be used for irrigation and exposed viscera should be covered or enclosed in plastic bags.
- Forced air warming devices and fluid warmers can be used in susceptible patients during surgery to prevent heat loss.

Can you tell me how forced air warming devices work?

They heat up the ambient air and pump it into a thin-walled channelled bag, which covers the patient as a blanket. The temperature of the air can be adjusted within a range of 32–40°C. It also has a thermostat which controls the temperature and prevents over-heating.

How can you warm intravenous fluids?

Two types of warmers are available. One is a dry-heat warmer and other is co-axial fluid warmer. The dry-heat warmer consists of two heating plates and a thin-walled polyvinyl chloride (PVC) bag is inserted between the plates. Intravenous fluids pass through the bag and get warmed. In a co-axial fluid warmer there is an outside tube which carries heated sterile water at 40°C and an inside tube which carries the intravenous fluid.

To what temperature do you warm the fluids? What happens if the temperature is too high?

Intravenous fluids and blood are normally warmed to 37°C. The maximum temperature to which the fluids can be warmed is 41°C. If the temperature is too high then blood can haemolyse, and it can also lead to hyperthermia.

Q3 The ECG

What is an ECG?

An electrocardiogram (ECG) is a surface recording of the electrical activity of the myocardium. It is recorded by connecting various electrodes through which electrical potentials are measured.

The display is recorded onto an oscilloscope or moving paper. The actual appearance of ECG depends on the position of electrodes in relation to the heart.

What are the components of an ECG monitoring system?

- Skin electrodes to detect the electrical activity of the heart.
- Amplifier to boost the signal.
- An oscilloscope or thin-film transistor (TFT) screen to display the amplified signal.

What are the components of an ECG electrode?

It consists of a silver:silver chloride electrode which is held in a cup and separated from skin by foam pad soaked in conducting gel. It has an adhesive flange which helps to keep the electrode in contact with skin.

Where do you place the electrodes for standard lead II?

Standard lead II is derived from negative electrode on the right arm and positive electrode on the left leg. The lead axes from three standard leads (lead I, II and III) form a triangle known as an Einthoven triangle.

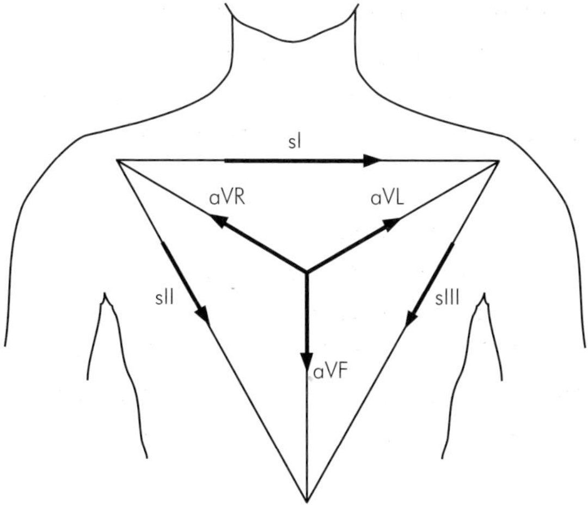

Figure 9.8 *Einthoven triangle*

What is a unipolar limb lead?

In a unipolar limb lead, the positive pole is attached to one of the limbs and the negative pole is attached to all three limb electrodes. The sum of the all three limb leads at all times is equal to zero potential. Thus the unipolar limb lead records the difference between an active limb lead and an indifferent electrode (zero potential) at the centre of Einthoven's triangle.

What potential risks may be associated with intraoperative ECG monitoring?

If the patient is improperly grounded, shocks or burns could occur as the electrodes complete a short circuit. New monitors have minimal risk because of patient isolation devices.

What artefacts can alter the ECG intraoperatively?

The following factors may lead to artefacts and inaccurate diagnosis:

- Loose or misplaced ECG wires or electrodes.
- Improper electrode placement or adhesion (hair, burned tissue, inadequate skin preparation, surgical scrub, dry-electrode gel).
- Motion, muscle activity (shivering, tremor, hiccupping, surgical preparation, diaphragmatic movement).
- Electrical interference can be either a 50 Hz (UK) mains line interference or due to high frequency from diathermy. Shielding of cables and leads, differ-ential amplifiers and electronic filters all help to produce interference-free monitoring.
- Patient contact by surgeons, nurses or other personnel.

What precautions do you take to avoid artefacts while attaching the electrodes?

Intended area of the skin should be prepared by gentle abrasion of the superficial epithelial layer with alcohol and cotton swabs. Hairy skin should be shaved. Wet and oily skin should be cleansed and allowed to dry. Whenever possible the electrodes should be placed over the bony prominences. Electrodes should be covered with water-resistant drapes if they are likely to be loosened by skin preparation solutions.

What precautions do you take to avoid artefacts from leads and cables?

Leads and connecting cables should be properly insulated. Lead and cable movements can lead to artefact, which can be minimised by twisting the leads on themselves.

Crossing of other monitoring cables (e.g. the SpO_2 cable) over the ECG leads will cause signal interference.

What other mechanisms can prevent artefacts?

The ECG monitors have filters to decrease environmental artefacts. Most ECG monitors have two modes. The monitoring mode has a frequency response of 0.5–40 Hz which eliminates both low and high frequency artefact and filters out baseline drift. This may distort the height of QRS and ST segments. The diagnostic mode has a wider frequency response of 0.05–100 Hz which is used to monitor S–T segment changes.

What is a differential amplifier?

A differential amplifier measures the difference between the potential from two sources. Any interference which is common to the input terminal (such as 50 Hz mains frequency) is eliminated. This rejection of common input frequency is known as common mode rejection.

What you mean by drift?

Variation in the output potential of an amplifier is known as drift. An amplifier contains semiconductor materials, the resistance of which varies with the temperature. Any change in the environmental temperature causes the direct current (DC) output potential to change.

What you mean by bandwidth of an amplifier?

The frequency range of an amplifier (when classified to a degree of accuracy over the distribution) is known as bandwidth. Interference can be avoided by correctly matching the bandwidth to the frequency of input signal.

What you mean by gain of an amplifier?

The ratio of the voltage at the output of an amplifier to the signal voltage at the input is known as gain. An amplifier should be suitable for the voltage range of the input signal.

What is the speed at which ECG is recorded?

ECG is recorded at a speed of 25 mm per second.

What voltage standardisation is used?

A height of 1 cm represents 1 mV.

Physiology 10

Key topics: clotting, immunology, fluid balance

Q1 Clotting

When you cut yourself what changes happen with respect to restricting the bleeding?

There are certain initial changes involving the blood vessel, platelets and plasma. The blood vessels constrict and the endothelium becomes procoagulant to form a potential base for the clots to form. The activated platelets adhere and aggregate. The plasma contributes to the fibrin formation.

Simultaneously, some inhibitory mechanism operates to limit the above changes and confine the changes to the site of injury.

Finally, when bleeding is controlled, the clot is removed by a process called fibrinolysis.

Tell me the steps involved in coagulation cascade.

Although there are differing opinions about the existence of two distinctive pathways, and other less specific mechanisms are now considered likely, classically they are described as intrinsic and extrinsic pathways. The extrinsic pathway is considered more important in normal in vivo coagulation response.

Can you explain the clotting mechanism?

Platelets form a primary haemostatic plug. They undergo adhesion, change in shape to enhance interaction between platelets, release their contents to enhance the clotting process and then aggregate. Loose aggregation of platelets in a temporary plug are bound together and converted into a definitive clot by fibrin. This

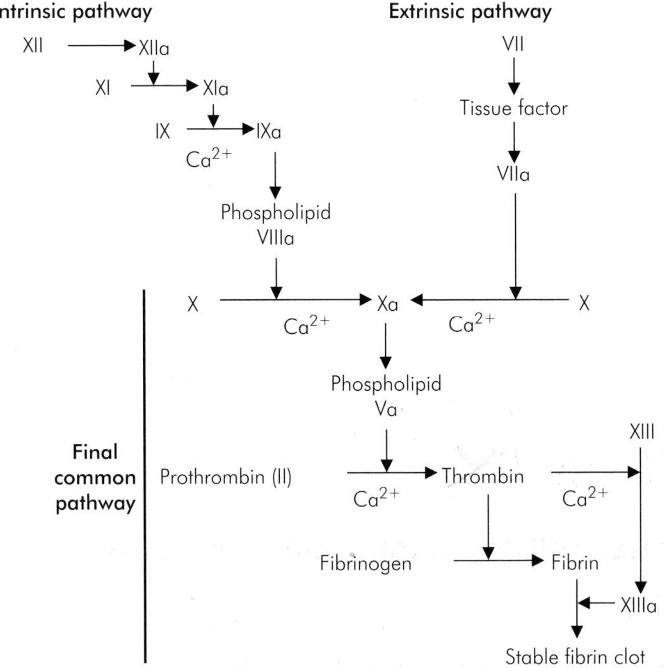

Figure 10.1 *Classical coagulation cascade*

involves a series of reactions in which fibrinogen is converted into a fibrin monomer which is then polymerised into fibrin.

What are the differences between intrinsic and extrinsic pathways?

The extrinsic pathway, as the name implies, needs 'tissue factor' for activation and this lies outside the vascular system. This tissue factor is a lipoprotein which activates factors VII. The extrinsic pathway is tested using prothrombin time (PT). The more standardised way of expressing the integrity of this pathway is international normalised ratio (INR). The extrinsic pathway is affected and hence PT is prolonged in warfarin administration, vitamin K deficiency, disseminated intravascular coagulation (DIC) and in liver disease.

In contrast, the intrinsic pathway is activated by substances present in the plasma within the vascular system. This is initiated by 'contact activation'. The cascade is initiated by activation of factor XII on exposure to certain surfaces. Activated partial thromboplastin time (APTT) is used to assess this pathway. Heparin therapy, DIC, and liver disease can affect this intrinsic pathway and hence prolong APTT.

Tell about the final common pathway. Where do the intrinsic and extrinsic pathways meet?

The final common pathway begins with activation of factor X to Xa which in turn will facilitate the conversion of prothrombin to thrombin in the presence of factor Va. Thrombin has a very important role in the coagulation pathway. It cleaves fibrinogen to fibrin. A revised coagulation hypothesis has highlighted a more extensive role of thrombin where thrombin returns back into the cascade and activates factors V and VIII. This step dramatically increases the efficiency of the system.

Thrombin time (TT) is useful in assessing the final pathway. Increasing use of the estimation of serum fibrinogen level has replaced routine testing of TT.

What are the naturally occurring inhibitors of coagulation?

Anti-thrombin III inhibits factors thrombin, Xa, XIIa, XIa and IXa by binding with them and forming inactive complexes. (Heparin acts by binding to anti-thrombin III and increasing its action).

Thrombin when bound to thrombomodulin (a thrombin binding protein, produced by endothelium), becomes an anti-coagulant.

Protein C and protein S are vitamin K-dependent factors. They inactivate Va and VIIIa.

The platelet aggregating effect of thromboxane A_2 is balanced by an anti-aggregate effect of prostacyclin.

A reduction in levels of these natural inhibitors can predispose to venous thrombosis.

Tell me how the fibrinolytic system works. What factors can enhance and inhibit fibrinolysis?

Thrombin and tissue type plasminogen activator (t-PA) activate the conversion of plasminogen into plasmin. Plasmin lyses fibrin and fibrinogen into fibrin degradation products (FDP).

Tissue type plasminogen activators streptokinase and urokinase enhance fibrinolysis.

Drugs such as aprotinin and tranexamic acid inhibit the action of plasmin and inhibits fibrinolysis.

In the laboratory setting, the fibrinolytic system is assessed using measurement of FDP and D-dimers.

Q2 Immunity

What do you understand by immunity?

Immunity is the ability to resist or overcome infection – a defence mechanism.

Can you name two types?

The two types of immunity are innate (natural) and acquired.

Acquired immunity is further classified into two types, humoral and cellular immunity.

Innate immunity does not require prior exposure to the offending agent. Complement system and macrophages are examples of this natural immunity system.

Acquired immunity requires lymphocytes, B lymphocytes for humoral immunity and T lymphocytes for cellular immunity. Acquired immunity needs prior exposure to the offending agent for an efficient response. Once 'memory' is gained, the system becomes very effective.

Humoral immunity is mediated by immunoglobins (produced by plasma cells, which are a differentiated form of B lymphocytes).

Cellular immunity is mediated by T lymphocytes. T cells produce lymphokines which have an important role in the immune response.

Tell me more about immunoglobulins.

Immunoglobins are circulating antibodies produced by plasma cells (found in the globulin fraction of plasma proteins). They contain four polypeptide chains, 2 long chains (heavy) and 2 short chains (light).

There are five classes: IgG, IgA, IgM, IgD and IgE.

What is their function? What exactly do they do?

- Neutralise protein toxins.
- Block the attachment of virus particles to the cells.
- Opsonise the bacteria.
- Activate the complement system.

When an immunoglobulin binds to an antigen there are several possible outcomes:

- An inactive complex may be formed, which will be phagocytosed.
- The antibody may act as an opsonin, thereby facilitating phagocytosis.
- The antibody may activate the complement system.

What is the complement system?

It is a system of complex plasma enzymes that mediate or regulate both innate and acquired immunity. This system is activated by two different pathways, classical and alternative:

1 *Classical pathway*: Immunoglobulins (IgG and IgM) bind to the antigen and the antigen–antibody complex activates C1. Eleven different enzymes are involved in this pathway (C1 to C9).

2 *Alternative pathway*: A circulating protein recognises the sugar residues in the bacterial/viral wall and activates C3. This pathway does not need the presence of any antibodies.

After a series of reactions C3a and C5a, the anaphylatoxins, are formed. They cause degranulation and release of histamine from mast cells, granulocytes and platelets causing local vasodilatation and hyperaemia.

What is a cytokine?

Cytokines are polypeptides (proteins) secreted by the cells of immune system that act as a soluble messenger of the immune system. They can be pro- or anti-inflammatory.

- *Pro-inflammatory*: TNF, IL-1, IL-6, IL-8, IL-12 and interferons
- *Anti-inflammatory*: IL-10, TNF-binding proteins.

What do you understand by cytokine balance?

In health, pro-inflammatory and anti-inflammatory cytokines are in balance.
This balance is upset by conditions such as trauma, sepsis and neoplasms.

What are the physiological functions of cytokines in the inflammatory response?

They upregulate adhesion molecules, which facilitates the adhesion of leucocytes to vascular endothelium.

On adhering to the endothelium, leucocytes release enzymes that degrade connective tissue such as endothelial basement membrane and endothelial junctions.

This leads to a leak of plasma proteins and oedema.

Q3 Fluid balance

Can you tell me what happens when you rapidly administer a litre of normal saline intravenously in an otherwise fit adult?

The changes can be analysed based on two different aspects:

1 The haemodynamic changes and the compensatory mechanisms.

2 How the body handles the excess fluid.

Rapid administration of a litre of normal saline causes significant increase in the circulating blood volume. The venous return increases, the cardiac output increases and there is an increase in the mean arterial pressure.The system tries to restore the normal blood pressure by immediate neural mechanisms and delayed humoral mechanisms.

The immediate neural mechanism involves the baroreceptors in the carotid sinus. Increased rate of firing from these receptors causes reflex inhibition of the vasomotor and cardiac centres in the medulla causing systemic vasodilation and a drop in the mean arterial pressure.

Later the humoral mechanism comes into play. The increase in the blood volume stimulates the low pressure–volume receptors which leads to a reduction in antidiuretic hormone (ADH) secretion from posterior pituitary. This causes diuresis.

There is a reduction in renin–angiotensin activity that in turn reduces aldosterone release, so that more sodium and water are excreted. This in due course will restore normal circulating volume.

Atrial natriuretic peptide (ANP) is released in response to atrial stretching following fluid overload. ANP will increase the glomerular filtration rate and the urinary sodium and water excretion. Vascular smooth muscle is relaxed and there is inhibition of plasma renin activity and aldosterone release.

As far as the distribution of the normal saline in the body is concerned, being isotonic it will tend to distribute within the extracellular fluid (ECF) compartment. ECF is made up of 3/4 interstitial volume and 1/4 intravascular volume. Therefore about 250 ml of the administered normal saline will eventually remain in the circulation.

What would be the response if it was blood or 5% dextrose instead of saline 0.9%?

When administered rapidly, the initial haemodynamic changes and the compensatory mechanism will be similar to that of normal saline. The distribution of the fluid within the various compartments varies. Blood tends to stay within the intravascular compartment.

5% dextrose is rapidly lost from the intravascular compartment. The glucose component is metabolised leaving 1000 ml of water. This equally distributes into the total body water (TBW). ECF being 1/3 of TBW, only about 333 ml remains in ECF. Of this 333 ml only 1/4 remain in intravascular compartment, which is about 84 ml.

Pharmacology 10

Key topics: adrenergic receptors, inotropes, suxamethonium

Q1 Adrenergic receptors and drugs

What are the types of adrenergic receptors? Where are they located?

The types include α- and β-receptors. α-receptors are subdivided into α_1- and α_2-, and β-receptors are subdivided into β_1, β_2 and β_3:

- α_1 is postsynaptic and is excitatory.
- α_2 is presynaptic and is inhibitory.
- β_1 is postsynaptic and is excitatory.

- β_2 is postsynaptic and is inhibitory.
- β_3 is postsynaptic and is associated with lipolysis and thermogenesis.

How do you classify sympathomimetic drugs?

They are classified according to their mechanism of action as direct-acting or indirect-acting sympathomimetics. Direct-acting sympathomimetics act directly via the adrenergic receptors. Indirect-acting sympathomimetics resemble norepinephrine and are transported by uptake into the nerve terminals. In the nerve terminals they displace norepinephrine.

They can also be classified depending on their structure as catecholamines and non-catecholamines. The basic structure of sympathomimetics is a benzene ring with amine side chains attached at C_1 position. A benzene ring with hydroxyl groups at 3rd and 4th positions is known as catechol. Sympathomimetics containing this basic structure are known as catecholamines. Catecholamines can be further classified as naturally occurring catecholamines and synthetic agents.

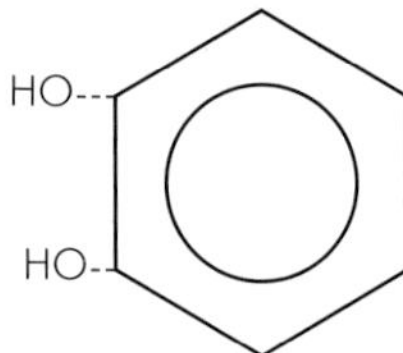

Figure 10.2 *Catechol ring*

- Catecholamines are dopamine, norepinephrine, epinephrine, dopexamine, dobutamine.
- Non-catecholamines are ephedrine, phenyephrine, turbutaline.

What are their clinical effects?

α_1-receptor stimulation produces vasoconstriction, relaxation of the smooth muscle of the gut, increased secretion of saliva and hepatic glycogenolysis. Stimulation of post-synaptic cardiac α_1-receptors causes a significant increase in myocardial contractility.

α_2-receptor stimulation inhibits release of autonomic neurotransmitters (mediates negative feedback which inhibits release of norepinephrine). It stimulates platelet aggregation.

β_1-receptor stimulation causes increased heart rate, increased myocardial contractility, relaxation of smooth muscle of gut, and lipolysis.

β_2-receptor stimulation results in vasodilatation, bronchodilatation, visceral smooth muscle relaxation and hepatic glycogenolysis.

Dopamine receptors: Stimulation of peripheral DA_1 receptors causes renal, coronary and mesenteric arterial vasodilatation and a natriuretic response.

DA_2 receptors are found in the basal ganglia and hypothalamus and are concerned with co-ordination of movements and inhibition of prolactin release.

Drugs acting on these receptors may cause agonism, antagonism or partial agonism and often have a mixture of effects on different receptors.

Table 10.1 *Drug–receptor interactions at adrenergic receptors*

	$Alpha_1$	$Alpha_2$	$Beta_1$	$Beta_2$
Agonists				
Norepinephrine	+++	+++	++	+
Phenylephrine	++	0	0	0
Clonidine	0	+++	0	0
Dopamine	+	0	++	++
Epinephrine	++	++	+++	+++
Dobutamine	0	0	+++	+
Salbutamol	0	0	+	+++
Isoprenaline	0	0	+++	+++
Antagonists				
Phentolamine	−−−	−−−	0	0
Phenoxybenzamine	−−−	−−−	0	0
Prazocin	−−−	−	0	0
Indoramin	−−−	−	0	0
Ergotamine	pa	−−	0	0
Labetalol	−−−	−	−−	−−
Propanolol	0	0	−−−	−−−
Atenolol	0	0	−−−	−

Note: +: agonist activity; −: antagonist activity; pa: partial agonist activity.

What are the neurotransmitters at the receptors of sympathetic nervous system?
In the sympathetic nervous system acetyl choline acts as a pre-ganglionic neurotransmitter and norepinephrine acts as post-ganglionic neurotransmitter.

Q2 Inotropes

What is an inotrope?
An inotrope is an agent which increases the force of cardiac muscle contraction.

Can you name some positive inotropic drugs?
They can be classified into three classes depending on their mechanism of action:

- *Class I*: Drugs that increase the intracellular calcium concentration (calcium, β-agonists, phosphodiesterase inhibitors, glucagon and digoxin).

- *Class II*: Drugs increasing the sensitivity of actomyosin to calcium – α-adrenergic agonists
- *Class III*: Drugs acting through the endocrine and metabolic pathways.

They can also be classified according to their affinity to the adrenergic receptors:

- Predominant β-agonists (dobutamine, dopexamine, isoprenaline).
- Predominant α-agonists (phenylephrine).
- Those with mixed α- and β- effects (epinephrine and norepinephrine).

When do you use calcium? What preparation do you use? What is the mechanism producing the inotropic effect?

Calcium is used to treat hypocalcaemia (when there is decreased ionised calcium in the blood) and to counteract the effects of high potassium.

Two intravenous preparations are available. Calcium gluconate 10%: 10 ml contains 9.3 mg of elemental calcium. Calcium chloride 10%: 10 ml contains 27.2 mg of elemental calcium. Either of these two preparations can be used but calcium gluconate requires three times the volume of calcium chloride.

An increase in cytoplasmic Ca^{2+} concentration facilitates binding of Ca^{2+} to troponin C. This causes movement of tropomyosin and reveals the actin binding sites for the myosin heads. This enables the myosin heads to attach themselves to actin filaments, which results in contraction of cardiac muscle.

What is the mechanism of action of epinephrine?

Epinephrine produces a dose-dependent stimulation of α- and β-adrenergic receptors. β-adrenoreceptors are coupled to Gs proteins that stimulate adenyl cyclase and increase the synthesis of cyclic AMP (cAMP). cAMP activates protein kinase which results in phosporylation of proteins leading to altered ionic permeability of cell membranes. This leads to increased Ca^{2+} influx into cells.

Epinephrine also activates α_1-receptors via Gq proteins. The enzyme phospholipase C is activated, which hydrolyses phosphatidylinositol biphosphate (PIP_2) into inositol triphosphate (IP_3). IP_3 increases the calcium influx into the cells.

Can you compare and contrast epinephrine with norepinephrine?

- *Structure*: Both are endogenous catecholamines
- *Mechanism of action*: Epinephrine predominantly stimulates β_1- and β_2-receptors at lower doses. At increasing doses it also stimulates α_1- and α_2-receptors. Norepinephrine has powerful α_1-adrenergic effects (it does have β_1-effects, but no clinically significant β_2-effects).
- *Pharmacokinetics*: Epinephrine is methylated by catechol-O-methyl transferase (COMT) into metanephrine which is then oxidised by monoamine oxidase (MAO) into vanillyl mandelic acid (VMA). Metanephrine is conjugated with glucuronic

acid or sulphates and excreted in the urine. Norepinephrine is taken up by the presynaptic neurons (uptake) and within the nerve terminal it is either recycled or metabolised by MAO. Outside the nerve terminals, it is also methylated by COMT into normetanephrine and vanillyl mandellic acid (VMA). Normetanephrine is conjugated with glucuronic acid or sulphuric acid and excreted in the urine.

- *Pharmacodynamics*: The cardiovascular effects of epinephrine are dose dependent. At low doses it produces increased cardiac output and coronary dilatation. The peripheral effects include decrease in systemic vascular resistance and fall in blood pressure. At low doses, through its β_2-effects it also causes splanchnic vasodilatation. At high doses α_1-effects predominate causing rise in systemic vascular resistance.

  Norepinephrine at low doses causes tachycardia but at higher doses it causes reflex bradycardia and splanchnic vasoconstriction. Systemically administered norepinephrine produces peripheral vasoconstriction and increase in both systolic and diastolic blood pressure. It may produce decrease in cardiac output and oxygen delivery due to increased afterload.

  Both these drugs increase the myocardial oxygen consumption. Norepinephrine causes reflex bradycardia and increases aortic root pressure which can partially compensate for increased oxygen demand.

Table 10.2 *Epinephrine and norepinephrine*

Properties	Epinephrine	Norepinephrine
Heart rate	++	−/+
Stroke volume	+++	++
Cardiac output	+++	0/−
Arrhythmias	++++	++++
Coronary blood flow	++	++
Systolic blood pressure	+++	+++
Mean arterial pressure	+	++
Diastolic blood pressure	+/0/−	++
Mean pulmonary arterial pressure	++	++
Total peripheral resistance	−/+	++
Cerebral blood flow	++	0/−
Muscle blood flow	+++	0/−
Skin blood flow	−−	−−
Renal blood flow	−	−
Splanchnic blood flow	−	0/−
Oxygen demand	++	0/+
Blood glucose	+++	0/+
Blood lactate	+++	0/+

Note: + = increase, − = decrease, 0 = no change.

- *Respiratory*: Epinephrine is a potent bronchodilator. Norepinephrine has no effects on bronchial tone. Both cause pulmonary vasoconstriction.
- *Metabolic effects*: Epinephrine increases basal metabolic rate and stimulates glycogenolysis. It also causes increased insulin and glucagon secretion. It increases Na^+ absorption from the renal tubules. Secondarily to its β_2-effect it increases the transport of K^+ into the cells. It increases oxygen consumption and may result in lactic acidosis.
- *Clinical uses*: Epinephrine is administered as a bolus in anaphylaxis and cardiac arrest. It is used as an intravenous infusion for its inotropic effects (0.01–0.5 μg/kg/min). It is also used as nebuliser to reduce upper airway oedema. Norepinephrine is mainly used to increase the systemic vascular resistance in refractory hypotension (as in sepsis).

What happens to the clinical effect of an infusion of epinephrine if it is used for 48 h? Why?

Response is reduced due to down regulation of receptors.

Q3 Suxamethonium

Can you draw the structure of suxamethonium?

Suxamethonium has a quaternary amine structure. Clinically it consists of two molecules of acetyl choline joined through the acetate methyl groups at their non-quaternary ends.

$$\left[CH_3-\overset{\overset{CH_3}{|}}{\underset{\underset{CH_3}{|}}{N^+}}-CH_2CH_2\,O-\overset{\overset{O}{\|}}{C}-C-CH_2CH_2-\overset{\overset{O}{\|}}{C}-O-CH_2CH_2-\overset{\overset{CH_3}{|}}{\underset{\underset{CH_3}{|}}{N^+}}-CH_3 \right]^{2\,Cl^-}$$

Figure 10.3 *Suxamethonium chloride*

How does suxamethonium act?

It binds to the nicotinic acetyl choline receptor and results in depolarisation of the motor endplate. Since the enzyme which hydrolyses suxamethonium is not present at the neuromuscular junction, it binds to the receptor for longer duration than that of acetyl choline (acetyl choline is rapidly hydrolysed by cholinesterase present in the neuromuscular junction). The persistent agonist effect at the receptor prevents the repolarisation of the end plate so it is refractory to further stimulation. As the suxamethonium diffuses from the junctional cleft, depolarisation occurs and muscle action potential is once again possible.

How is suxamethonium metabolised?

It is rapidly hydrolysed by plasma cholinesterase (pseudocholinesterase) to succinyl monocholine and choline. Pseudocholinesterase has a large capacity to hydrolyse suxamethonium, so that only a small amount (10–20%) of the administered drug reaches the neuromuscular junction. Succinyl monocholine is further hydrolysed into choline and succinic acid. Neuromuscular block produced by suxamethonium is terminated by its diffusion away from the neuromuscular junction. Administration of 1 mg/kg of suxamethonium results in complete suppression of response to neuromuscular stimulation in approximately 60 s. In patients with normal plasma cholinesterase level the neuromuscular block usually lasts for 4–6 min.

What are the side effects of suxamethonium?

- *Myalgia*: This is more common in young female, ambulatory patients following minor surgery. It is secondary to the damage produced in muscles due to unsynchronised contraction during fasciculations.
- *Parasympathetic effects*: Sinus bradycardia is more commonly seen in children and after repeated doses.
- *Hyperkalaemia*: A raise in serum potassium by about 0.5 mmol/l has been seen in normal individuals. Severe hyperkalaemia may be seen in patients with severe metabolic acidosis and hypovolaemia. An exaggerated hyperkalaemic response is also seen in patients with burns, major trauma with muscle injury, patients with neuromuscular disease and patients with paraplegia. Burns patients are at risk from 24 h after the injury and for up to 18 months.
- *Increased intraocular pressure (IOP)*: The increased IOP is manifested within 1 min of injection and lasts for about 6 min. The mechanism has not been clearly defined, but it is known to involve contraction of tonic myofibrils and transient dilatation of choroidal blood vessels.
- *Increased intragastric pressure*: This is presumed to be due to fasciculations of abdominal muscles. As the lower oesophageal sphincter tone also increases, normally there is no increased risk of regurgitation. However in certain situations where the lower oesophageal sphincter mechanism is altered (in pregnancy, abdominal distension due to ascites, hiatus hernia and bowel obstruction), there may be increased risk of regurgitation.
- *Suxamethonium apnoea*: Recovery from suxamethonium induced neuromuscular block is dependent on plasma cholinesterase. A prolonged neuromuscular block after suxamethonium can be due to both acquired and genetic factors.
- *Malignant hyperpyrexia*: It is a trigger for malignant hyperpyrexia. Masseter spasm has been observed after administering suxamethonium but this is not consistently associated with malignant hyperpyrexia.

- *Tachyphylaxis and Phase II block (dual block)*: Decreased response may be observed with repeated doses and this may precede the gradual development of phase II block (change of characteristics of block into a non-depolarising block). This is most commonly seen when large doses or prolonged infusions are used.

What is the dibucaine number? What is dibucaine?

Dibucaine (cinchocaine) is amide local anaesthetic that inhibits normal plasma cholinesterase. Dibucaine number is defined as the percentage of enzyme inhibition produced by dibucaine using benzylcholine as a substrate. Under standardised test conditions dibucaine inhibits the normal enzyme by 80% and abnormal enzyme by 20%. This percentage inhibition is known as the dibucaine number. Dibucaine number indicates the genetic makeup of plasma cholinesterase enzyme, it does not measure the concentration of the enzyme in the plasma, nor does it indicate the efficiency of the enzyme in hydrolysing suxamethonium.

Table 10.3 *Dibucaine number*

Genotype	Incidence	Dibucaine number	Response
Eu: Eu (homozygous typical)	96%	80	Normal
Eu: Ea (heterozygous typical)	4%	60	Mildly prolonged (10–20 min)
Ea: Ea (homozygous atypical)	1:2800	20	Prolonged (4–8 h)

Can you name some drugs which can cause inhibition of plasma cholinesterase?

- Cytotoxic drugs (methotrexate).
- Local anaesthetics (lidocaine and amethocaine).
- Anti-cholinesterases (ecothiopate eye drops, neostigmine, edrophonium and organophosphorous compounds).
- Others (lithium, ketamine and metoclopramide).

What is role of suxamethonium in current anaesthetic practice?

Despite of many adverse effects suxamethonium is still in clinical use due to its rapid onset of action, short duration and profound depth of neuromuscular blockade. It is still the drug of choice for rapid sequence induction. It produces optimum condition for tracheal intubation within 30 s.

Clinical 10

Key topics: diabetes, obesity, failure to regain consciousness, spinal anaesthesia

Q1 A 40 year old obese (BMI = 39) male patient is scheduled for incision and drainage of peri-anal abscess. He is a known diabetic controlled with oral hypoglycaemic drugs.

How would you proceed?

Perform a complete pre-operative assessment of this patient to includes history, clinical examination and investigations with special reference to diabetes mellitus.

On clinical examination he appears dehydrated. Heart rate is 120/min, respiratory rate is 30/min and blood pressure is 110/60 mmHg. Heart sounds are normal and chest is clear.

What investigations would you like to do?

Investigations should include full blood count (haemoglobin, white cell count, platelets), urea and electrolytes, blood glucose, Glycosylated haemoglobin (HbA1c) and electrocardiogram. Further investigations will be dictated by the history and examination findings.

His blood glucose is 26 mmol/l. Would you like to do any other investigations?

Yes. A blood gas analysis should be taken to check the acid–base status. Also ask for analysis of urine sample for ketone bodies.

On arterial blood gas analysis pH is 7.20 and urine is positive for ketone bodies. What is your diagnosis?

The picture is suggestive of probable diabetic ketoacidosis.

What is the significance of measuring HbA1c?

Glycosylated haemoglobin (HbA1c) measurement is the most widely used measure of long-term glycaemic control over 6–8 weeks period.

What is the normal value of HbA1c?

It should be less than 7%.

How is HbA1c formed?

HbA1c is produced by glycosylation of the N-terminal valine of the beta-chain of haemoglobin.

The level of HbA1c depends upon:

- Red cell lifespan.
- Prevailing blood glucose concentration.

Providing red cell lifespan is normal, HbA1c measures mean blood glucose concentration over the preceding 60 days (i.e. half-life of red cell).

What are the complications of diabetes?

Complications of diabetes can either be acute metabolic derangements or chronic organ damage.

- *Metabolic*: Diabetic ketoacidosis, non-ketotic diabetic coma, hypoglycaemia, hypokalaemia, dehydration.
- *Cardiovascular*: Ischaemic heart disease, myocardial infarction and cardiomyopathy.
- *Neurological*: Cerebrovascular accident, peripheral neuropathy, autonomic neuropathy: orthostatic hypotension, resting tachycardia, cardiac arrhythmias, altered bowel and bladder habits.
- *Renal*: Diabetic nephropathy.
- *Eyes*: Retinopathy.
- *Gastrointestinal tract*: Gastroparesis (predisposition to aspiration).
- *Musculoskeletal*: Stiff joint syndrome (predispose to difficult intubation).
- *Immune system*: Impaired or delayed surgical wound healing.

Why are you concerned about anaesthetising a diabetic patient? What are the problems?

There is a definite interaction between surgery and diabetes. Both pre-operative fasting and the stress response related to surgery can adversely affect glucose metabolism. Patients with diabetic ketoacidosis will have significant acid–base disturbance, and fluid and electrolyte imbalance. Diabetic patients have an increased co-morbidity. All these factors can lead to increased perioperative morbidity and mortality.

This patient's body mass index (BMI) is 39. Can you comment on this?

He is morbidly obese.

What is BMI?

Body mass index (BMI) is a measure of obesity that takes into account patient's height and weight. It is defined as weight (kg)/height^2 (m).

BMI $<$ 18.5: Underweight
BMI 18.5–24.9: Normal range
BMI 25.0–29.9: Overweight
BMI 30.0–34.9: Obesity
BMI 35.0–39.9: Morbid obesity
BMI $>$ 40: Severe morbid obesity

What are the problems associated with obesity?

Problems can be broadly classified into physiological, anatomical and those due to altered pharmacokinetics:

- Physiological:
  - *Respiratory system*: Total respiratory compliance is decreased mainly due to a reduction in chest wall compliance. It can be as little as 30% of normal. Functional residual capacity (FRC) and expiratory reserve volume (ERV) are reduced. FRC can fall within the closing capacity and therefore result in alveolar collapse. These patients have increased CO_2 production and increased O_2 consumption. In order to maintain normocapnoea minute ventilation increases. With increasing obesity, alveolar ventilation is insufficient to excrete CO_2, hence $PaCO_2$ increases (obesity hypoventilation syndrome). These patients often have obstructive sleep apnoea.
  - *Cardiovascular*: There is increased cardiac output and left ventricular wall thickness increases due to extra cardiac workload. There is an increased incidence of ischaemic heart disease, hypertension, cardiomegaly and congestive cardiac failure.
  - *Gastrointestinal*: Increased gastric acidity and fluid volume, hiatus hernia (increased risk of aspiration during induction) and fatty infiltration of liver may all be seen.
  - *Endocrine and metabolic*: An increased incidence of diabetes and hypercholesterolaemia.
  - *Musculoskeletal*: Osteoarthritis and limited mobility are associations with obesity.
- Anatomical:
  - Such patients often have a short and fat neck, limited movement of atlanto-occipital joint, large size of chin, breasts and thoracic fat. All these factors can lead to difficult airway both for mask ventilation and endotracheal intubation.
  - Difficult venous cannulation, difficult to locate anatomical landmarks for invasive monitoring procedures and regional anaesthesia techniques may present problems. Problems should be anticipated with non-invasive blood pressure measurement which may be inaccurate.
  - Difficulty in positioning may dictate special arrangements for the operating table.
- Pharmacokinetics:
  - Compared to total body weight obese patients have a smaller proportion of total body water and a greater proportion of body fat. These factors change the proportion of drug distributed to various body compartments (e.g. increased uptake of volatile agents into and delayed elimination from the fat

compartment). Fat soluble drugs (benzodiazepines, thiopental) will have an increased volume of distribution. Increased levels of lipoproteins affect drug protein binding. Renal excretion and hepatic excretion of drugs can also be reduced. Relative overdosage can occur when drug dose is calculated based on actual weight of the patient.

What complications may you encounter during the post-operative period in obese patients?

- *Immediate*: Delayed recovery and effect of residual anaesthetic agents. Respiratory depression leads to hypoventilation and desaturation in the recovery room. Upper airway obstruction is common and in patients with associated obstructive sleep apnoea it can be severe.
- *Delayed*: Respiratory complications include atelectasis, chest infection and eventual respiratory failure. Delayed wound healing, wound infection and deep vein thrombosis are more likely in these patients.

How would you manage this patient?

Aim is to control the blood glucose and correct the dehydration, electrolyte and acid–base imbalance. This patient is best managed in a high dependency unit with invasive monitoring. An arterial line will prove useful for monitoring arterial blood gases and electrolytes. Airway, breathing should be assessed and supplemental oxygen should be administered. Conscious level, fluid intake and urine output should be monitored.

For the control of blood glucose, a short acting soluble insulin infusion should be started as per a sliding scale regimen. The aim is to maintain the blood glucose between 4–8 mmol/l. Once the blood glucose is less than 12 mmol/l, 5% dextrose infusion is started at a rate of 125 ml/h.

Serum potassium should be monitored every hour and hypokalaemia is corrected.

Since the clinical signs are suggestive of dehydration, 1 l of sodium chloride 0.9% should be administered intravenously rapidly. Further administration of fluid will be guided by clinical parameters, central venous pressure and urine output.

Why does serum potassium level decrease during insulin infusion?

Insulin also increases the permeability of many cells to potassium, magnesium and phosphate ions. The effect on potassium is clinically important. Insulin activates sodium–potassium ATPase in the cells, causing a flux of potassium into cells. Under certain circumstances, injection of insulin can kill patients because of its ability to acutely depress plasma potassium concentrations. Therefore frequent monitoring and supplementation of potassium during insulin infusion is important.

For example, the concentration of the oxygen in the pulmonary veins is 200 ml/l and in the PA is 150 ml/l, so each litre of blood going through the lungs takes up 50 ml of oxygen. At rest, the blood takes up 250 ml/min of oxygen from the lungs. Hence Cardiac Output = 250/50 = 5 l.

$$M = Q \times (A - V).$$

Therefore, $Q = M/(A - V)$.

Here M is VO_2, A and V are CaO_2 and CvO_2 respectively. VO_2 is the oxygen uptake over 1 min, CaO_2 is the oxygen content of arterial blood and CvO_2 is the oxygen content of the venous blood.

Thus, cardiac output = $VO_2/(CaO_2 - CvO_2)$.

How can you measure oxygen taken up by the lungs (oxygen uptake)?

The subject is asked breathe through a spirometer filled with 100% oxygen, with carbon dioxide absorption system. Oxygen taken up over a minute can be calculated by knowing the final oxygen concentration at the end of 1 min.

How do you measure the arterial and venous oxygen content?

A mixed venous sample is obtained from the PA catheter and oxygen content is calculated. An arterial sample is obtained and the oxygen content of peripheral arterial sample is assumed to be equal to oxygen content in the pulmonary veins.

Tell me about the indicator dilution techniques in cardiac output measurement.

The indicator can be a dye or temperature change.

- *Dye dilution*: A known amount of dye (indocyanine green) is injected into a central vein, and its concentration in the peripheral blood is measured continuously. The change in indicator concentration over time is measured, a curve is achieved which is re-plotted semi-logarithmically to correct for recirculation of the dye. A computer calculates the area under the dye concentration curve and derives the cardiac output.

  The dye should be non-toxic and should rapidly mix with blood. Indocyanine green is suitable due to its low toxicity and short half-life.
- *Thermodilution*: This is the most commonly used invasive method to measure the cardiac output at the bed side. 5–10 ml cold saline is injected through PA catheter into the right atrium. Temperature changes are measured by a distal thermistor of a PA catheter. A curve similar to dye dilution is obtained by plotting the temperature changes over time. An analogue computer calculates the cardiac output using the Steward–Hamilton equation. Cardiac output is inversely proportional to the area under the temperature–time curve.

What does PiCCO stand for? What are its advantages?

PiCCO stands for Pulse induced contour cardiac output.

This method uses a standard central line with a temperature sensor on the distal lumen and a thermodilution sensor arterial catheter, placed in either the femoral or brachial artery. This is a much less invasive method and reduces the risk associated with the insertion of a PA catheter.

Although the thermodilution curve is longer and flatter than in traditional PA thermodilution it is not influenced by the respiratory cycle. The algorithm used computes left ventricular stroke volume by measuring the area under the systolic part of the waveform from the end of diastole to the end of the ejection phase and dividing the area by the aortic impedance. This calculation provides a measure of stroke volume.

It also estimates Intrathoracic blood volume (ITBV) and Extravascular lung water (EVLW). Changes in ITBV have been shown to correlate well with changes in cardiac output and may be a more appropriate monitoring parameter for cardiac preload. EVLW gives a measure of water content in the lungs and is a guide to fluid management in shock.

Q2 Soda lime

Why do you use the circle breathing system?

The circle system is used to facilitate recirculation of expired gas after removal of carbon dioxide. It reduces fresh gas flow (FGF) requirements and hence minimises atmospheric pollution. It also helps to humidify and warm inspired gas.

What chemicals are used to absorb carbon dioxide in the circle system?

Soda lime or baralyme are used in the circle system to absorb carbon dioxide from the expired gas.

What is the composition of soda lime?

Composition by weight (%):

NaOH	5
Water	14–19
Silica	0.2
$Ca(OH)_2$	Approximately 80

Sodium hydroxide improves the reactivity of the mixture. Silica is to prevent the disintegration of granules, but is not required with the modern manufacturing process.

An indicator is added which changes the colour when active constituents exhausted. Colour changes can be pink to white or white to violet depending on the indicator dye.

What is the size of soda lime granules? Why is that important?

Size of granules is 4–8 meshes. A strainer with 4 meshes has four openings per inch.

They are also manufactured as spheres of 3–5 mm size. In UK the granules are supplied to a British Pharmacopoeia (BP) standard of 3–10 mesh size.

Index